Traditional Medicine System in India

In December 2010, the Mission organized a seminar on manuscripts related to Indian traditional medicine system at ORIML, University of Kerala. The seminar dealt with different aspects of Ayurveda and its importance to modern society. The main focus of this seminar was on Ayurveda practiced in Kerala, the state which has its own ethnic style of Ayurvedic treatment.

The seminar gave ample opportunities to the experts to put forth their views and share their research-oriented knowledge with others.

Samīkṣikā Series
No. 6

General Editor
PRAFULLA KUMAR MISHRA

The Samīkṣikā Series is aimed at compiling the papers presented by the various scholars during the seminars organized by the National Mission for Manuscripts. The seminars provide an interactive forum for scholars to present to a large audience, ideas related to the knowledge contained in India's textual heritage.

In keeping with the title, the Samīkṣikā (research) Series is concerned with research papers of distinguished scholars and specialists in different intellectual disciplines of India.

Traditional Medicine System in India

Edited by

K.G. Sreelekha

National Mission for Manuscripts

Dev Publishers & Distributors

Published by:
National Mission for Manuscripts
Indira Gandhi National Centre for the Arts
11 Man Singh Road
New Delhi 110 001
Phone: 91 11 2307 3387
E-mail: directornamami@nic.in
Website: www.namami.nic.in

and Co-published by:
Dev Publishers & Distributors
2nd Floor, Prakash Deep,
22, Delhi Medical Association Road,
Darya Ganj,
New Delhi-110002
Phone : 011-43572647
e-mail: devbooks@hotmail.com
website: www.devbooks.co.in

ISBN 81–904029–8–6 (Series)
ISBN 978–93–80829–06–7
First published 2014

Contents

Foreword vii

Preface ix

Key to Transliteration xi

1. Āyurveda Netra Cikitsā with Special Reference to Keralīya-cikitsā-paddhati—*N.P.P. Namboothiri* 1
2. Pharmacology and Pharmaco Therapeutics of Ayurvedic Drugs—*P.R. Jaya* 17
3. Bālaciktsā—An Introductory Study—*Rejani. R. S.* 27
4. Bālatantra Manuscript—A Study—*R. Girija* 37
5. A Critical Study of Agastya—Yogasāram Kilippaṭṭu—*Lalu S. Kurup* 41
6. Interpretation, Adaptation and Translation—Process of Pratisaṃskaraṇa—*K. Muthulekshmi* 45
7. Vaidyaka Manuscripts in the Oriental Research Institute and Manuscripts Library, Thiruvananthapuram —*P.L. Shaji* 53
8. Āyurveda—A Vibrant Tradition of Kerala—*K.G. Sreelekha* 59
9. Nayanavithi Vākatam—*Kum. Radha* 67
10. Poison Treatment/Anti-Dote Treatment in Tamil Palm-leaf Manuscripts—*Senthil N.* 75
11. Rediscovering the Unique Tradition of Gynaecology and Obstetrics in Kerala Based on Manuscripts—*P. Vasumathy* 85

12. Systems of Medicine in Tantra Manuals of Kerala—*S.A.S. Sarma* 103

13. Tamil Medical Manuscripts in the Oriental Research Institute and Manuscripts Library, Thiruvananthapuram—*O. Padmakumari* 115

14. Textbook Tradition of Āyurveda—*Vinod Kumar* 121

15. Toxicology in Āyurveda—*N. Sam* 149

16. Uses of Herbal Medicine—*P. Prema* 153

17. Varma as Therapy—*T. Mohana Raj* 159

18. Vikṛti Vijñjāna-Samkṣepa: Impish Knowledge-Concise—*Saramma Varghese* 165

Contributors 171

Foreword

Indian system of treatments and application of medicine are as old as the age of Ṛgveda. Lord Śiva was addressed as doctor of doctors. भिषक्तमं त्वां भिषजां वृणोम्यहम्. He was also the doctor who applies only water. There was only medicine of herbs/औषध, which is medically used even today. But in the process of evolutions the introduction of rasāyana/रसायन alchemy by Nāgārjuna; the great Buddhist sage brought revolution in Indian medicine. The use of mercury in as early as fifth century AD (by Nāgārjuna-रसरत्नाकर and रसलक्ष्यपुट) in unbelievable even today; when alchemy is a developed science.

Kerala has developed a lot in the domain of traditional treatment which is known as शुद्धचिकित्सा. Manuscripts thereof are plentily available. The manuscripts of मातङ्गलीला in Trivandrum Library is quite interesting for the treatment of elephants. Moreover मर्मलक्षणम् for acupressure and texts like सहस्रयोगम्, चिकित्सायञ्जरी, धाराकल्पम्, वैद्यमञ्जरी, योगामृतम्, सन्निपातचिकित्सा are quite striking and they deserve to see the light of the day.

Besides the interesting texts in Tamil there are thousands of Ayurvedic texts available all over the country. They are kept with the families of traditional practitioners of medicines.

Not only that there are many types of treatment by different strata of the society. It is curious to note that like Buddhists, Nāthayogis have developed तैलचिकित्सा where application of oil is important. Al these types of treatment brought together shall prove how rich our country is without any insurance etc. for treatments. The most important aspect of these texts are; that, the treatment is within the reach of any ordinary person vis-a-vis in the age of costly treatment of corporate world.

PRAFULLA KUMAR MISHRA
Director

New Delhi
20th May, 2014

Preface

The Oriental Research Institute & Manuscripts Library is a department of the University of Kerala, which has crossed its centenary. This department was born out of tutelary interests since the Kings of Travancore were always patrons of art and literature. Ours is the second largest collection of its kind in Asia and there are around 65,000 works out of which around 3000 are Ayurveda Manuscripts.

India is a country which is full of medicinal plants and famous for indigenous medicine system. This system of indigenous medicine prevailed in India in times when modern medicine was not emerged. The famous Ayurvedic physicians Charaka & Susruta lived in India and Vagbhatan is believed to have been lived in Kerala and he wrote Ashtangasamgraha and Ashtangahridaya, which are still considered to be basic texts of Ayurveda in Kerala. Kerala is a state which has its own ethnic style in Ayurvedic treatment which has been found to be the most effective compared to other parts of the country. Now Ayurveda has emerged as a stream in the study of medicine which is considered to be as good as modern medicine. Ayurveda is preferred by people since it has got no side effects and hence becoming more and more important day-by-day. It provides cure for almost all kinds of diseases including terminal diseases.

Hence our attempt through this National Seminar on 'Manuscripts related to Indian Traditional Medicine System' is to probe into the different aspects of Ayurveda and its importance in the modern society. We are hoping that the deliberations and discussions will throw light into many hidden areas which have not become so popular; but needs attention.

I take this opportunity to thank all scholars who contributed the seminar us in response to our invitation. My sincere gratitude goes to National Mission for Mauscripts for all the support rendered to us. Special thanks goes to Dr. Sangamitra Basu, Co-ordinator, Publication for her cooperation in publication of this volume. I also express my gratitude to the Hon. Vice Chancellor & Kerala University authorities for their support.

DR. K.G SREELEKHA
Project Co-ordinator ORIML MRC &
Prof. & Head, ORI & Mss. Library,
University of Kerala, Kariavattom

New Delhi
14th May, 2014

Key to Transliteration

VOWELS

अ a	आ ā	इ i	ई ī	उ u	ऊ ū
(but)	(palm)	(it)	(beet)	(put)	(pool)
ऋ ṛ	ए e	ऐ ai	ओ o	औ au	
(rhythm)	(play)	(air)	(toe)	(loud)	

CONSONANTS

Guttural	क ka	ख* kha	ग ga	घ gha	ङ ṅa
	(skate)	(blockhead)	(gate)	(ghost)	(sing)
Palatal	च ca	छ cha	ज ja	झ jha	ञ ña
	(chunk)	(catchhim)	(john)	(hedgehog)	(bunch)
Cerebral	ट ṭa	ठ* ṭha	ड/ड़ ḍa	ढ*/ढ़ ḍha	ण* ṇa
	(start)	(anthill)	(dart)	(godhead)	(under)
Dental	त ta	थ tha	द da	ध dha	न na
	(path)	(thunder)	(that)	(breathe)	(numb)
Labial	प pa	फ* pha	ब ba	भ bha	म ma
	(spin)	(philosophy)	(bin)	(abhor)	(much)
Semi-vowels	य ya	र ra	ल la	व va	
	(young)	(drama)	(luck)	(vile)	
Sibilants	श śa	ष ṣa	स sa	ह ha	
	(shove)	(bushel)	(so)	(hum)	
Others	क्ष kṣa	त्र tra	ज्ञ jña	ळ* l	ॠ* ṝ
	(*kṣātriya*)	(*triśūla*)	(*jñānī*)	(play)	

अं ( ) *ṁ* or *ṃ amusūra* (nasalisation of preceding vowel) like *saṁskṛti/or soṃskṛti*

अः *visarga* = *ḥ* (aspiration of preceding vowel like (*prātaḥ*)

ऽ *Avagraha* consonant #' consonant (like-*imé vasthitā*)

Anusvāra at the end of a line is presented by m (म्) and not *ṁ*

*No exact English equivalents for these letters.

1

Āyurveda Netra Cikitsā with Special Reference to Keralīya-cikitsā-paddhati

N.P.P. Namboothiri

Introduction

Though we are here to preview Netra-cikitsā we should remember that Āyurveda understands body as a whole. So systemic approach is given due respect along with specific localized eye treatment.

Importance of Netra

- Situated in Ūrdhvāṅga
- Importance of Ūrdhvāṅga (in the context of *roga-mārga*)
- *Madhyama roga-marga.*

Sarvendriyāṇāṃ nayanaṃ pradhānam

cakṣuḥ pradhānaṃ sarveṣāmindriyāṇāṃ vidurbudhāḥ/
dharaṇīhārayuktānāṃ jyotiṣāmiva bhāskaraḥ//
—*Śuśrata-saṃhitī*

Eye is the most important among sense organs. It is as important to human being as sunlight is to earth.

Netra rogas:

- Vātaja = 10

- Pittaja = 10
- Kaphaja = 13
- Raktaja = 16
- Sannipātaja = 25

Most of the *sannipātajas* are *sarakta-Sannipātaja*

Striking note

- *Rakta* is a palpable presence while enumerating *netra rogas.* In case of *abhiṣyanda* it is having a specific role.

Abhiṣyanda

prāyeṇa sarve nayanāmayāstu bhavanti
abhiṣyanda-nimittamūlāḥ

—*Suśruta-saṃhitā, Uttaratantra*

This is where the *rakta* gets the importance.

Abhiṣyanda is played in the pool of *rakta* so *Abhiṣyanda* is very important in understanding, diagnosing and managing almost all *netra rogas.*

Cikitsā

Bringing imbalanced *doṣas* back to normalcy (*doṣa- sāmya*); in *netra* context its managing *abhiṣyanda,* i.e bringing hormonious balance between *uṣṇa* and *śīta* or *pitta* and *kapha* is the main aim of *cikitsā*

Aim of Āyurveda:

svasthasya svāsthyarakṣaṇam/
āturasya vikārapraśamanaṃ ca//

Aim of Kriyākalpa:

netraprasādana
netra-roga-śamanārtha

Sāma Lakṣaṇa

udīrṇavadanaṃ netraṃ rāga-dveṣa-samanvitam/
gharṣaniṣṭhodaśūlāsrayuktām āmānvitaṃ viduḥ//
—Aṣṭāṅgahṛdaya, Sūtra

In *āmavasthā* of *netra, āścyotana, piṇḍī, seka, vidalaka* are the procedures to be advised.

Nirāmalakṣaṇa

nirāmāvasthā mandavedanatā
kaṇḍuḥ samrambhastu prasannataḥ/

—

Aṣṭāṅgahṛdaya, Sūtra

praśāntavartmatā cakṣnou
sampaktvaṃ gadamādiśet

(Com.)

By looking into the *praśasta lakṣaṇa* of *vartma,* one can judge the *nirāmavasthā.*

Treatment Modalities

In total, classical texts explain seven *kriyā halpas*

- Āścyotana
- Seka
- Piṇḍi
- Vidalaka
- Añjana

- Tarpaṇa
- Puṭapāka

Āścyotana

sarveṣāmakṣirogāṇām ādau āścyotanaṃ hitaṃ/
rukthoda kaṇḍū-gharṣaniṣṭhoda dāharāga-nibarhaṇaṃ//

—Ibid., 23.1

Indication: All *sāmāvasthā* of *netra.*

All treatment for eye starts with *aścyotana* if *āmāvasthā* is perceived.

- Triphala, yaṣṭhi, utpala—Pittaja
- Stanya—bleeding conditions of eye
- Lodhra kaṣāya—vātaja and sannipātaja
- Sigrupatra svarasa in kaphaja
- Sphaṭika, karpūra drops as prasādana

Piṇḍī

yuktabheṣajakalkasya piṇḍī ca kavala-mātrayā/
vastrakhaṇḍena sambadhya netre abhiṣyandanāśinī//

—

Bhāvaprakāśa

netrābhiṣyanda-yogyā sā vraṇeṣvapi nibadhyate/

(sā.u.)

Guḍūci Kumārī Piṇḍī—Pittaja abhiṣyanda

Vidalaka

Vidalako bahirlepo netrapakṣmavivarjitaḥ/

(*Sa.U.13*.30).

Avyakteṣvevaṃ guṇameva pakṣmaparihāreṇa
akṣikośālepanam

—*Aṣṭ. Sūtra* 32/2.

Indications and Duration

utpannamātre taruṇe netraroge vidalakaḥ/
kāyo dāhopadehāśru śopha-roganivāraṇaḥ//
—*Carakasaṃhitā, Cikitsā.* 26.231

tasya mātrā parijñeyā mughālepa vidhānavat/
(*sa.u.*13.30)

Durvādilepa—Durvā, Yava, Sārivā, Gairika, Ghṛta in Pain and Redness

Añjana

vyaktarūpeṣu doṣeṣu śuddhakāyasya kevalā/
netre eva sthite doṣe prāptamanjanamācaret//
—*Śuśrutasaṃhitā, Uttaratantra*

- Hemanta and Śiśira—Afternoon.
- Grīṣma and Śarat—Morning
- Varṣā—not cloudy and not in early morning
- Vasanta—Always

Vilvādi Gulika
Nārikela Rasakriya Añjana

Añjana Bheda:

According to Action

1. Lehana
2. Ropaṇa
3. Prasādana
4. Snehana

According to difference in form

1. Guṭikā—Mahābala *roga*
2. Rasakriyā—Madhyamabala *roga*
3. Cūrṇa—Hīnabala *roga*

Examples

- Candanādi añjana
- Paśupatāñjana
- Nakulāñjana
- Timirāñjana
- Garuḍāñjana
- Mukulāñjana

Añjana

Disposal rate is minimum, Tissue contact time is more.

Maximum absorption—

Acts as subconjunctival injections and also permeable there through sclera and acts on posterior segment disorders.

Tarpaṇa

When to do?

āture śānta rāgāśru śūla-samrambha-dūṣake/
nivāte tarpaṇam yojyaṃ śuddhāya ūrdhvakāyāya//

When not to do ?

Contra-indication

durdinātyuṣṇaśīteṣu citāyāsa-bhrameṣu ca/
śāntopadrave cākṣṇoḥ tarpaṇaṃ na praśasyate//

Absorption is very high as drugs are lipid, soluble penetration is high irrespective of molecular size.

Drug vehicle and bio availability:

Tissue contact time and bioavailability is highest and significant therapeutic concentrations are achieved.

Disposal: drug is retained for a prescribed period of twenty minutes (average)

Puṭapāka

- *Puṭena pākaḥ puṭapākaḥ*
- *mṛdādikapākadvayena nirmiti ca auṣadha pāka/*

Types

- Snehana—200 MK (3 minutes)
  Animal Fat Kakolyādi gaṇa dravyas etc.
- Lekhana—100 MK (½ minute)
  Honey, Māṃsa Bhasmas of gold silver and copper
- Prasādana—300 MK (4 minutes)
  Milk and Ghee, Tikta Ropaṇa dravya

Compliance:

Duration—1 to 3 days
Quantity—25 ml each eye
Disposal
Absorption same as in *tarpaṇa*
Tissue contact time and bioavailability is also same as *tarpaṇa.*

Seka	Chronic and severe affections of the eyes
Āścyotana	First line of treatment in ocular inflammatory conditions. Rāga, Dāha, Aśru-srāva, Śopha,Toda
Piṇḍī/Kavalikā	Netra abhiṣyanda and Vraṇas
Vidalaka	Inflammatory conditions, Congestion, Redness, Irritation
Añjana	Pakva Avastha of Netra, Alpa Śopha, Atikāṇḍū, picchilatā, Alpāśru srāva, Alpa-rāga. After-Śarīra-Saṃśodhana and Āścyotana
Tarpaṇa	Jīhyata, Tamyata Rukṣata, Pakṣma Śata, Kṛconmilana Adhimantha, Timira , Arjuna, Śukra, Abhiṣyanda, Śakṣākṣipāka, Śotha, Vātaviparyaya, Śirotpāta.
Puṭapāka	Same as Tarpaṇa. After Tarpana to increase the dṛṣṭībala.

Special treatment modalities

- *Tala*
- *Talaputhachil (śirolepa)*

- *Jalaukāvacaraṇa*
- *Lekhana*
- *Kizhisvedana*
- *Annalepana*
- *Eye massage*
- *Bandhana*
- *Mūrdhni tailam (pichu, abhyaṅga, dhara, śirovasti)*
- *Takradhārā*

Tala

- Keeping medicated paste over bregma

Eg : Vasa, lakṣa, yasṭhi, triphala with vasa svarasa in bleeding eyes

Jalaukāvacaraṇa

- Will be good in recurrent stye, kṛmigranthi, scleritis, śiraharṣa and śirotpāta.

Lekhana

Scraping gently with japā mukula or samudraphena in the palpebral conjunctiva

Eg .In follicular conjunctivitis ,

Kizhisvedana

- It is called avaguṇṭana sveda in classics
- Eg. Ciñcā and haridrā svedanam is effective in stye, allergic conjunctivitis
- Yava sveda before tarpaṇa in some cases .

Annalepana

- Apply navara paste and doing gentle circular massage
- Good in weakness of eye lid, degenerative myopia, ROP

Eye Message

Apply medicated oil over eye lid and do gentle massage

Very effective in vātāhata vartma, high myopia, amblyopia

Bandhana

- After keeping jāti puṣpa or specific paste (sigrutvak) and doing bandhana for specific time period
- In keratoconus, after tarpaṇa, puṭapāka, and in eye injuries.

Mūrdhni Taila

- *PICU*
- *ŚIRO ABHYANGA*
- *ŚIRODHARA*
- *ŚIROVASTI*

Takradhārā

- As a śamana procedure
- Rūkṣaśīta prayoga
- Best in handling *pitta raktaja abhiṣyanda*
- Kledaharaṇa.

Eg:

- Diabetic retinopathy
- Glaucoma

Management of Complex Eye diseases

ARMD

Treatment Plan (*Yukti*)

Macular/Retinal function simulates to that of ālocaka Pitta (Cakṣu vaiśeṣika).

Old age macular degeneration, dry type should be treated on the line of vāta dominating pittaja.

Wet/neovascular type should be treated on the line of pure pittaja disease.

Treatment

- Virecana with Trivṛt ghṛta, Daśamūla ghṛta
- Saptāmṛta loha, Śatāvaryādi cūrṇa, Āmalaki cūrṇa

- Vasanta kusumākara rasa, Śuddha vaṅga (ca. compound), Ārogyavardhani vaṭi, Basantamālini laghu
- Bhallātaka rasāyana
- Dhanadarasnādi kaṣāya, Pathyakṣadhatryādi kaṣāya

DIABETIC RETINOPATHY

Treatment Plan

Largely aimed at prevention and strict metabolic control of:

- blood sugar
- blood pressure
- dyslipidemia

This reduces the progression of diabetic retinopathy.

Medicines for Glycemic Control

- Samīra pañcaka kaṣāya
- Niśākatthakādi kaṣāya
- Niśāmalaki yoga
- Katthaka khadirādi kaṣāya
- Phala trikādi kaṣāya
- Vara cūrṇa

Medicines for control of blood pressure

- Āśvangandhā cūrṇa
- Śaṅkhapuṣpī svarasa
- Daśamūla kaṣāya
- Rudrākṣa
- Parthāṛṣta
- Punarnavādi kaṣāya
- Pravala Bhasma

Medicines for Dyslipidemic control

- Varanādi kaṣāya
- Rasanādi kaṣāya

- Trayodaśāṅga guggulu
- Kaiśora guggulu
- Citrakādi vaṭi
- Ārogyavardhanī rasa
- Rasa Sindūra and its compounds

Exercise and Yogi kriyā

- Ardhamatsyendrāsana
- Madhukāsana
- Kapāla Bhāti Prāṇāyāma
- Uttāna padāsana
- Anuloma Viloma Prāṇāyāma
- Vāhya Prāṇāyāma
- Sarvāṅgāsana

External Therapies

- Takradhārā with vasa guḍucyadi kaṣaya
- Āścyotana with Vinayakāñjana
- Piṇḍī with Āmalaki leaf, guḍuci leaf or vasa leaf
- Añjana with Candanādi añjana
- Netradhārā with dārvyādi kṣīra kaṣāya
- Tarpaṇa with Jaḍaveda ghṛta

EALE'S DISEASE

Treatment plan

- Eale's disease seems to be like that of Parimalayī timira-pitta raktaja disease.
- Virecana with Triphalā ghṛta, Ārogyavadha compound and pitta hara treatment.

Treatment of Rakta-Pitta

- Samīra pañcakam kaṣāya
- Guḍūcyādi kaṣāya
- Drākṣādi kaṣāya
- Netrarakṣa kaṣāya

- Saptāmṛta loha

RETINITIS PIGMENTOSA

Normally treated at four stages
- Kapha viṣama dṛṣṭi
- Kapha vidagdha dṛṣṭi
- Kaphapittavidagdha dṛṣṭi
- Dṛṣṭi hata

.30–40 % manageable
Purely Rasāyana Cikitsā

Steps:

Śodhana Cikitsā
Bṛṃhaṇa Cikitsā

Treatment
Śodhana cikitsā involves
- Snehana with Vidaryādi ghṛta, Vainateya ghṛta or Mahātriphala ghṛta
- Virecana with Avipattikara cūrṇa

Bṛṃhaṇa Cikitsā involves
- Śamana kaṣāyas like Dhanada rasanādi, Samīrapañcaka, Netrarakṣā etc.

External applications like
- Añjana with nakulāñjana, Āścyotana with mahāpadma ghṛta, Seka with kaśyapa kaṣāya
- Tarpaṇa with Jātaveda ghṛta, Kaśyapa ghṛta.
- Śirodhārā with Śaśāṅka taila
- Picu with mahādaśamūla taila, bhujaṅga patra taila
- Śirovasti with bhujaṅga patra taila
- Puṭapāka with svarasa

Treatment is aimed at

- Relieve discomfort
- Provide smooth optical surface
- Prevent structural corneal damage
- Restoration of natural tear film

Local

- Āścyotana with Drākṣā, Candana processed and filtered out of Taṇḍulodaka . Honey alleviates lacrimation and burning.
- Irrigation of eye with cold unboiled milk with a bit of Saindhava.
- Añjana prepared from Śūṇṭhī rubbed with Ghṛta and Stanya.
- Kaśāñjana.
- Nasya with Kṣīrabala taila or Anu taila.
- Tarpaṇa with Jīvantyadighṛta, Kaśyapa ghṛta
- Puṭapāka with puṭapāka svarasa.
- Oral Ghṛta-pāna after meals, jīvantyādighṛta, Mahā-triphala ghṛta and Kaśyapa ghṛta.
- Vasti with milk processed in Madhuka, Śatāvahā, Ghṛta.

KERATOCONUS

- *Vāta* and *Rakta* seem to be major pathological factors.
- Structural changes are said to occur in superficial type of *vāta–rakta* by Ācārya Caraka.

Line of treatment

Preventive : Antenatal and Postnatal

Vāta and Rakta vitiating diet and requirements to be avoided

- Nutritious diet along with specific emphasis on liver functions
- Vasti cikitsā
- Gudućī, Āmalaki, Madhuyaṣṭi, Śatāvari, Milk, Ghee, Śāli Cāval, Māṅsa rasa.

Curative:

Following line can be adopted as ocular therapeutic measures from Vāta-Rakta Cikitsā (*Caraka Saṁhitā*)

- Blood letting
- Śodhana-Snehana–Virecana
- Repeated Anuvasana and Niruha Vasti.
- Pariśeka, Pradeha (Vidalaka)
- Food and Ghee made out of non-irritant drugs
- Superficial type of vāta rakta should especially be managed by ālepa (Vidalaka), abhayaṅga, pariṣeka, upanaha (Piṇḍī)

MYOPIA

- Ususally treated in the line of prathama-paṭalagata-timira

Treatment

- Snehapana with vainateya ghṛta, mahānīla ghṛta, kaśyapa ghṛta
- Virecana with Avipattikar cūrṇa
- Nasya with Anutaila, Kṣīrabala twenty-one Āvartī
- Internal kaṣāya with Netrarakṣa kaṣāya, Ākśabījādi kaṣāya, Dhanadarśādi kaṣāya, Samīrapañcaka kaṣāya
- Āñjana Candanadī, Mukulāñjana, Sunetra
- Āścyotana
- Āñjana ghṛta,vinayakāñjana
- Seka with Kaśyapa kaṣāya
- Eye massage with Kṣīrabala twenty-one Āvartī and Mahākukkuṭamāṅsa taila
- Śirodhara with Śaśāṅka taila,Bhujaṅgapatra taila, Aśvagandhā taila
- Picu with Bhujaṅga patra taila, Śaśāṅka taila
- Annalepana
- Eye exercise

- Tala with Bhujaṅgapatra taila
- Tarpaṇa with Mahānīla ghṛta,Triphala ghṛta, Ananta ghṛta

GLAUCOMA

- Treated in the line of Adhimanda
- In open angle glaucoma śīta and stambhana is done
- In closed angle glaucoma svedana, recana and sroto viśodhana are employed
- Treatment
- Snehapana with Thriphalādi ghṛta,Tilaka ghṛta, Vainateya ghṛta
- Virecana with Avipattikara cūrṇa, triphala cūrṇa with triphala kaṣāya, Nimbvamṛtādi eraṇḍa
- Nasya with Anu taila
- Śirodhara with Śaśāṅka taila, Guggulutiktaka taila
- Śiro Vasti with Śaṣāṅka taila

2

Pharmacology and Pharmaco Therapeutics of Ayurvedic Drugs

P.R. Jaya

Āyurveda is a science coming down from the Vedic period. It is an Upaveda of Atharvaveda. Ṛgveda also mentions the practices of Āyurveda.

It comprises the philosophy of life. It was the only mainstream health care system in early periods. It is one of the traditional medical system of Kerala.

The definition of health/Āyurveda

It is the equilibrium of *doṣas, dhātu, mala* and *kriyā* and the purity and clear status of *ātman* (soul), *indriya* (sense organs) and *manas* (mind) which is *āroyga.*

Life can be defined as the combination of *śarīra* (body), *indriya* (sense organs), *sattva* (*manas*) and *ātman* (soul).

The universe is based on the pañcamahābhūtas, viz. ākāśa, (space), pṛthvī (earth), vāyu (air), jala (water) and agni (fire). The Ayurvedic system says that the body is also *pañcabhāutika* and the medicines i.e. plants and animals are also *pañcabhautika.* So the *pañcabhautika śarīra* can be treated with *pañcabhautika* drug.

The basic units of *śarīra* are comprised of three elements known as *tridoṣas.* They are *vāta, pitta* and *kapha.* They are also *pañcabhautic. Vātakadoṣa* is *ākāśa* and *vāyu bhūta* predominant, *pitta* is *agni* and *jala* predominant and *kapha* is *jala* and *pṛthvī* predominant. So treating with *pañcabhautika* drugs is a necessity to passify the *rogāvasthā* of a person.

The four *pādas* or factors to make a treatment perfect are:

1. *Bhiṣak*: Vaidya-doctor
2. *Dravya*: drugs
3. *Paricāraka*: bystander/helper
4. *Rogī*: Patient

If these four pādas perfectly merge the treatment will be a success.

Drug/*dravya* is an important component. A perfect *dravya* had again four qualities as mentioned

1. Bahukalpana i.e. which can be made into many formulation;
2. Bahuguṇa with many properties;
3. Sampannatā is the wealth of drug with *rasa* (taste), *Guṇa* (qualities), *vīrya* (potency), etc.
4. Yogyatā is the correct selection of drug to be used in the apt situation.

The drug/*dravya*, if is properly used it is equivalent to *amṛta* (nectar) and if improperly used it is like *viṣa* (poison). *Nāma* (name), *rūpa* (morphology) and *guṇa* (quality) of medicine should be known properly.

Ayurvedic medicine are of different types. They can be used as single drugs, i.e. plants, metals and mineral drugs and animal drugs used in a single. It can be used as formulations also, i.e. a herb with a mineral or animal one and vice-versa. Herbo-mineral, herbo-animal and mineral – animal preparations can be used. All the three in combination is also a drug of choice. On this basis the source medicines are mentioned as *jaṅgama* (animal product) *udbhida* (herbs) and *pārthiva* (minerals).

Ayurvedic medicinal preparation and formulation are many in number.

1. *svarasa*: which is the expressed juice of herbs
2. *kalka*: grounded paste of medicine and when they are dried known as *cūrṇa* (powder)
3. *kvātha*: peapared *kaṣāya*
4. *yavāgu* and *yūṣa* are juices of dhānya or cereals
5. cold *kaṣāya* and hot *kaṣāya*
6. tablets and capsule
7. semi-solid *lehya* preparation
8. fermented preparation like *ariṣṭas*
9. mineral drug preparation.

The treatment principle of Āyurveda is addition to the body with same properties as that of *doṣas* and *dhātus* when they are of decreased level in the body. Deletion of the defected *doṣas* and *dhātus* with opposite properties when they are of excess in body.

Pharmacology

Pharmacology is the branch of medicine or biology that deals with the action of drugs and pharmacotherapeutic is the study of therapeutic uses and effects of drugs in the body.

The Ayurvedic view of pharmacology and pharmacotherapeutics of Āyurveda drugs are as follows. According to it *dravya* or drug is comprised of *rasa, vīrya, vipāka, prabhāva* and *karma*

According to modern pharmacology also, the drug actions are based on tanin, resin glycosides, essential oils, volatile oil and alkaloid, present in them.

Rasa: taste

They are six in number. They are *madhura* (sweet), *amla*

(sour), *lavaṇa* (salty), *kaṭu* (spicy), *tikta* (bitter) and *kaṣāya* (astringent). The different parts of the tongue can perceive the tastes and it makes effect on the body, whether it is a food or medicine or a level of medicines.

Guṇas: properties and qualities of drugs/*dravya.* Guṇas are forty-one in number. It includes twenty *śārīrika guṇas* which are present in medicines also.

Vīryas: potency is mentioned as two in number though eight numbers are mentioned. But all these eight potencies come under two, i.e. hot and cold. Hot potency is fully controlled by sun and cold potency is controlled by moon.

Vipāka: is post digestive taste. They are three in number. i.e. *madhura, amla* and *kaṭu.* After digestion the sweet and salty food and medicine convert to *madhura* v*ipāka*; sour food to *amla vipāka;* bitter and spicy food to *kaṭu vipāka.* From these three *vipākas, tridoṣa,* will be produced. From sweet *kapha doṣa,* from *amla* (sour) *pittadoṣa* and from spicy (*kaṭu*) *vātadoṣa* is produced.

Prabhāva can be mentioned as:

a. Serendipity, i.e. a propensity for making fortunate discovers while looking for something else;
b. Empirical, derived from or guided by experience or experiment
c. Or it can be mentioned as an effect of a drug which is magical or unexpected
d. Through the rasādibhāva a different drug action is observed and that is *prabhāva.*

Karmas: it is what these drugs do in the body. fifty *karmas* mentioned by Caraka and twenty-two by Śārṅgadhara.

Karma: pharmcotherapeutics is the targetted action of a drug and it includes pharmacokinetics and pharmacodynamics.

The *rasa, guṇa* and *vīrya* of the drug explains the pharmacology of Ayurvedic drugs.

The *vipāka, prabhāva,* and *karma* of the drug explain the pharmcotherpeutics of a drug.

Of these the detailed explanation of *śarīrika guṇas* and *karma* is essential.

Śārīraka guṇas are twenty in number.

There are ten guṇas with their opposite guṇas which are mentioned below:

1. Guru–Laghu heavy-light
2. Mantha–Tīkṣṇa/dull sharp
3. Hima–Uṣṇa/cold–hot
4. Snigdha–Rūkṣa/oily–dry
5. Ślakṣma–Khara/smooth-rough
6. Sāndra–Drava/dense-liquid
7. Mṛdu–Kaṭhina/soft-hard
8. Śthira–Cala/static-mobile
9. Śūkṣma–Sthūla/subtle-gross
10. Viśada–Picchila/clear–cloudy

These *guṇas* are also *pāñcabhautika* and they have specified action on the body

Guṇas	*Bhūtas Predominant*	*Actions*
Guru	earth, water	building/bṛṅhaṇa
Laghu	fire, air, ether, space	reducing/laṅghana
Śīta	water	Cooling/stambha
Uṣṇa	agni	healing/svedana
Snigdha	water	Moistening/kledana
Rūkṣa	earth, fire, air	absorbing/śoṣaṇa
Mantha	earth, water	slowing/pacifying/ śamana
Tīkṣṇa	fire	penetrating/purifying/ śodhana

Guṇas	*Bhūtas Predominant*	*Actions*
Sthira	earth	stabilising/dharṇā
Cala	air	stimulating/preraṇa
Mṛdu	water	loosening/sladhana
Kaṭhina	earth	hardening/dried
Viśada	fire air ether (space)	Cleansing-Kṣalana
Picchila	earth, water	Adharing-lepana
Ślakṣṇa	earth, water	healing/ropaṇa
Khara	air	scraping/lekhana
Sūkṣma	air, space	pervading/vivaraṇa
Sthūla	earth	covering/samvaraṇam
Sāndra	earth, water	solidifying/prasādana
Drava	water	liqufying/vilodana

Out of the forty-one *guṇas,* above are twenty guṇas, another ten parādi *guṇas,* are as follows

1. para–superior
2. apara-inferior
3. yukti–method of using/rationale
4. saṅkhyā–enumeration
5. saṃyoga/vibhāga–combination/diversion
6. pṛthaktva–separateness
7. parimāṇa–measures
8. saṃskāra–processing
9. abhyāsa–repeated use

The other five *guṇas—śabda, sparśa, rūpa, rasa,* and *gandha* which attribute to the perception of sense organs. The molecular level impact of medicines on sense organs can enhance or counter act the effect of treatment.

The last six *guṇas* are *ādhyātmika guṇas.* They are *buddhi* (intelligence), *icchā* (like), *dveṣa* (dislike), *sukha* (happiness), *dukha* (sorrow), and *prayatna* (effort). The pharmacology of drugs depends on the emotional or psychological status of a patient and is expressed through these guṇas.

Ācārya Caraka gives fifty *karmas* or actions through fifty groups of drugs with ten each. Drugs with similar action are combined together and mentioned as *mahākaṣāya yoga.* Śārṅgadhara's drug action view is with more of modern perspective.

The fifity *mahākaṣāyayoga karmas* with examples are quoted below:

1. Jīvanīya–helps to protect life and enhance longevity. They are vitalizing agent, eg. Jīvanti, liquorice etc.
2. Bṛṁhanīya–bulk promoting drugs which increase body weight and helps in the formation of new cells like kurunthotti or bala.
3. Lekhanīya–reducing agent–reducing fat mustha
4. Bhedanīya–breaking agent, breaks, accumulated one, eg. vacā
5. Sandhyānīya–healing agents-aloe vera
6. Dīpanīya–digestive stimulants–pippali
7. Balya–tonics like śatavarı
8. Varṇya–enhance complexion–mañjiṣṭha
9. Kaṇṭhya–Benfefical for throat–drākṣā
10. Hṛdaya–heart foric–dāḍima (pomegranate)
11. Tṛptighna–anti saturative, e.g. Rasna
12. Arśoghna–anti haemorrhoidal, e.g. Kuṭaja
13. Kuṣṭhaghna–antidermatitis, khadira tree
14. Kaṇḍughna–anti pruritc like nīmbu
15. Kṛmighna–anti helmenthic like vidang
16. Viṣaghna–anti toxins or counter poison like turmeric, tulasī
17. Stanya janana–lactogogogne–promotes secretion of milk e.g. vidari
18. Lacto depurants–purify breast milk, e.g. guḍuci

19. Śukra janan–spermatogenic–increase sperm count–e.g. Aśvagandhā
20. Śukrashodha–sperm purifying–removes toxins from sperm, eg. Kuṣṭa

21–27 are adjuvant groups of drugs and used in Pañcakarma therapy

21. Snehopaga–drugs boosting oleation of the body
22. Svedopaga–boosting sudation therapy
23. Varmaṇopaga–help in emetic therapy
24. Virechanopaga–helps in purgative therapy
25. Āsthapanopaga–helps in boosting kaṣāya vasthi and matra vasthi
26. Anuvāsanopaga–helps in boosting kaṣāya vasthi and mātrā vasthi
27. Śirovirecanopaga–drug action to help in nasya–nasal dropping treatment
28. Chardinigraha–antiemetic–ginger
29. Tṛṣṇānigraha–thirst reliever and hydrate tissues–nimbu (lemon)
30. Hikkānigraha–stops hiccop–ela

31-35. Related with *mala* (stool) and *mūtra* (urine) *vegas* (urges). Colour to mala and mūtra by purīṣa virajanīya and mūtra virajanīya group of drugs
- to stop the passing of excess mala and mūtra by purīṣa saṁgrahanīya and mūtra saṁgrahanīya drugs
- to make urge of mūtra by mūtra virecanīya drugs

36-37. Kāsahara and svāsahara drugs relives cough and breathlessness like kanṭakarī, vasa.

38. Śotha hara–relieves oedema or swelling–punarnava, trikanṭaka.

39. Jvarahara–which relieves fever or pyrexia–mustha, kiratatikta, parpadaka

40–43. Śramahara–to relieve exhaustion, dāhapraśamana–to relieve thirst of body, udardapraśamana–to relieve allergic rashes of the body, śītapraśamana–to relieve–red pigmented rashes of body

44-45. Aṅgamardapraśamana–relieve bodyache, e.g. Karpūra, śūlapraśamana–relieves colic, hiṅgu (asafoetida)

46-49. Śoṇitsthāpana–stopping the blood flow, e.g. Lodhra
Vedanasthāpana–Pain killer–guggullu
Saṁjasthāpana–boosts brain function–brāhmī
Prajasthāpana–make firm the fertilised e.g.–vidari, bala

50 Vayasthāpana–rejuvenate the body and promote longevity, e.g. abhaya, dhātrī (Indian gooseberry). From vitalising agent to rejuvenating agent, 50 formulations of 10 drugs–each is mentioned.

Śārṅgadhara gives following actions of drugs:

1. Dīpana–enhances agni or digestive fire
2. Pācana–enhance digestion
3. Dīpa Pācana–both the above factors
4. Śamana–balances the imbalanced doṣas
5. Anulomana, śramaśamana, bhedana, recana–these four groups of drugs act on malāśaya and due to the function of laxation to purgation.
6. Vamana–śodhana, chedana, lekhana, grahi, sthabhana, rasāyana, vyavayī, vikaśī, madakarī, prāṇahara, pramadī, abhiṣyandī, all these groups of drugs are having specific function of the body.

Effect of drug

The effect of drug is primarily due to the grace of God. Mahāvaidya or God designs it.

The other factors are—how the drug is collected, the time of collection, whether clean and from auspicious part it is collected, the month in which it is collected, place of collection of drugs and purpose of collection. The dosage, time and route of administration of medicine also speak out the efficacy. The mind and attitude of *Vaidya* and *rogī* also important in efficacy.

Through *daśavidha parīkṣā, āsthana parīkṣa, pañcendriya parīkṣā, trividha parīkṣā,* etc. the patient is examined thoroughly and then the correct choice of medicine is advised seeking the *roga prakṛti* and *rogi-avasthā.* The quality drug is administered in correct quantity and apt compounding and is thereafter dispensed for its intake. The drug generates effects on body by above-said ways and disease is pacified. The pharmacology and pharmacotherapeutics of Ayurvedic drugs bear vast scientific knowledge which needs to be taken seriously for inter-disciplined reserarch.

3

Bālaciktsā—An Introductory Study

Rejani. R. S.

Āyurveda, the science of life, prevention of diseases and instrumental of longevity is the oldest and most holistic medical system available on the planet today, which was the contribution of India to the world. Origin of Āyurveda which has flourished through generations cannot be determined as it continued either in practice or from mouth to ears. The origin of Āyurveda can only be tied up with either myths or epics, other than this it is impossible to find out a particular time of origin for Āyurveda. Āyurveda holds a predominant position in Indian subcontinent. Alleviation of diseases and retaintion of health are the aims of Āyurveda.

More than a treatment methodology, Āyurveda deals with our routine lifestyle. The ancient wisdom of this healing system was a part of the spiritual tradition of the Sanātana Dharma (Universal Religion), or Vedic Religion. "Anything that are related to our life is a matter of concern in Āyurveda. . That is why no other branch of science holds this immensity as Āyurveda do." These are the words of Padmabhooshan K. Raghavan Thirumulpadu.

Medication in Āyurveda is still based on the prescriptions in the *Carakasaṃhitā*, the *Suśrutasaṃhitā* and the *Aṣṭāṅgahṛdaya.* But according to the geographical features and availability of medicines there is a practice that they had made the contents of the books contemporary. That means the treatments are made in to practice in accordance with the timely needs. Based on this custom treatment, methodology differs from place to place.

In Kerala Āyurveda had achieved a great popularity even from the ancient times. Its magnificence reached to its apex during the period from 5th to 8th century AD, that is along with Buddhism. In other words Buddhist monasteries were also used as Āyurvedic Centres. Traditional medicinal systems were also popular in these monasteries. Some medicinal systems in Kerala were also included in this. For example *svedana, virecana, vamana,* etc.

For convenience of treatment Āyurveda can be broadly classified into eight sections. They are Kāyacikitsā, Bālacikitsā, Rasāyanacikitsā, Ūrdhvāṅgacikitsā, Śalyacikitsā, Viṣacikitsā, Vājīkaraṇacikitsā, etc. Each one of them has its own respective heritage in Kerala, especially for Bālacikitsā and Viṣacikitsā. Considering the significance of Bālacikitsā in Āyurveda, *Bāla-chikitsā—an introductory study* has been selected as the subject for this paper.

The Bālacikitsā is a section among the medicinal books that are kept in Kerala University Oriental Research Institute and Manusctripts Library. There are thirty-three books in the library on this subject. Out of these thirty are manuscripts and the remaining are transcripts. The source of this paper is the transcript under the register number 1201.

When we study the ancient books on this subject, an understanding about how they analysed the matters and arrived at conclusions is inevitable. Commonly in the books dealing with the Bālacikitsa often follows the subsequent procedure, i.e. garbhakāla cikitsā, prasavakāla cikitsā, bālyakāla cikitsā. But this book gives more importance to Bāla-cikitsā than Prasava-cikitsā. Now we can have a glance at the peculiarities of the content of this book.

Familiarization of the symptoms for various diseases forms the basis of diagnosis. This familiarization followed by examination determines the treatment methodology. This thinking formulates the following method in the book; first it tells us about the symptoms of various diseases then a description about the symptoms followed by treatment methodology and then about the preparation of medicines. For example we can look in to a particular context in this book

> *"janikkummattudarathil munnam janica pillaikku mathīva kānam pādadikesam vranamai bhavikkum samichu kolvan pani pāramundam dwarangal thorum vranamai bhavikkum kesum kozhinjeedu matheeva vegal adāramayullava roga chihnam".*

Then about treatment methodology.

> *"Pavittu Vachoru Kashsyamum nannādou kodukkamithu kerathailey poyidumennalithukondu melle pokaikilammaikku chikitsa venam"*

Then it tells about the preparation of medicine. Let us look into it later. This is the structure of this book. We can now see the other characteristics of this book. The book begins with offering prayers to both deities and guru (teacher).

> *"gurunadhanenikkettam thunayaivarikeppozhum*
> *Kavimathumithauvannam kadalvarnanumadaral*
> *Gurupādayugam chithe maruveeduka santhatam*
> *Piriyathe vasikkenam kripaya gunavaridhe".*

It is quiet common in ancient books, that it begins with offering prayers to gods. This book also follows the same manner and then it describes about various diseases for children.

Bālacikitsā speaks about the cause and medication for various infirmities that the children from infants to those who are below sixteen years go through. In the first chapter it briefly introduces the diseases that are common to the children. Ācārya finds that there are two reasons for infirmities that happen to the children. One of the reasons is *bālagrahapīḍās* and the other one by *bhūta-preta–piśācas.* Āyurveda consider *bālagrahadevatāprīti* and mantras or tantras for curative purposes. Ācārya believes that above all these by performing *dāna-dharma* and performing offerings to gods we can maintain a healthy lifestyle. According to the modern science religious beliefs are included as it will create a positive energy in human beings. It may be the reason that our Ācāryas recorded this earlier. For example let us look into a *pratipadya.*

> *"Balapeedakal chollunnu vibudadikal munname*
> *Balagṛhangal ennonnundu peedippanoru devatha*
> *Oroothingalkkathoronnu perumoronnathai varum*
> *Balikarmangalum veere chikitsayumathanganey".*

This means that saints had already told about the *bālapīdās.* There is a category namely *Bālagrahangal.* Each one of these grahas has its own devatā and name. They have different *balikarmas* and treatments also.

The Ācārya does not forget to advice the physicians too.

> " *vannu chonnalavarkkorupayadikal chollanam*
> *Paropakaram cheyyanam vridha thanneyumadaral*
> *Phalasiddhi bhavicheedum mattoredathu sammadhal*
> *Sidhaushadangaloronne sidhamayittirikkanam*
> *Pānalepanamayittum balikarma vidathilum.*

This means that patients must be treated with reasons. It must be done respectfully. For that purpose physicians must learn the medicines by heart. By mentioning that the knowledge he had acquired from his teacher is made useful to the public by means of this book he concludes the first chapter.

Second chapter deals with the preparation of medicines for the diseases related with head. The preparation of ointment for the heat effecting the head due to *acne* is then mentioned.

1. Athikkai, ellu and thumbappoovu are with milk and then and mixed it with butter and when is applied to the head it alleviates the illness.
   Preparation methods of more than one medicines and ointments for a particular disease is stated by Ācāryas.
2. The ointment for acnes that are formed in our ears is prepared by mixing vettalian koodu, aratha, chukku together along with loose curd.
3. For puss formed in our ears, juice of thulasi leaves are mixed with coconut oil and then is added with vayambu, kanjirakkambu, kunthirikkam and induchoodam and it is prepared by boiling. The resultant drops can be used as medicine.
4. When redness and swelling happens to child's eyes, honey mixed with the juice of Poovamkurunnila can be applied as drops to heal the disease.

The author following the Ācāryas then describes the medication for dysentery. In older days dysentery and vomiting are the main reasons for the death of children. Even elders used to lose their immunity power and suffer by dysentery. Hence Ācāryas describe about the medication for dysentery in the most suited way. There are a number of medicines for dysentery but some selected ones are taken as examples.

1. Kottatholi boiled with loose curd (moore) can be taken as medicine for dysentery.
2. Jathikka mixed with curd is also a good medicine for dysentery.

Karappaṇ/pyoderma: It holds a prime position in communicable diseases that are affecting the children. Eighteen of its kind are mentioned in this book. Preferred medicines are mentioned below. Ācārya warns that generally for all types of Karappaṇ, oil and ghee must be omitted. After that medicines for different types of karappaṇ are prescribed.

1. *chorakkarappaṇ:* bandhooka pushpam, thechippoovu are mixed with loose curd and then the mixture is cooked and then filtered and can be applied.
2. *chenthekarappaṇ:* root skin of thechi mixed up with coconut milk and can be applied frequently for this disease. This medicine is useful for all types of pyoderma/ karappaṇ.
3. *Neerkkarappaṇ:* ulli, thippali, elathari and mulaku mixed with murukkila rasam can be taken as medicine for neerkarappaṇ.
4. *Pannikkarappaṇ:* kodalurukki veru, kattu mulaku kodi, thandu and njarinjil

The Ācārya did not forget to prescribe the preparation of syrups for pyoderma.

Akakkarappaṇum akamundikkum koodi mukkidikku:

Juice of Amarayila, koorkkayila and pacha manjal are mixed with per 100gm of induppu, narunadillizhangu, veluthulli boiled and has to be taken two times daily. It is an excellent medicine for all the eighteen types of pyodermas.

Likewise it describes the preparation of medicine that can be applied to head for the children suffering from pyoderma.

For example: elathari, elavangatholi, muthanga kizhangu, puli njarambu, kurunthotti veru and vayambu together taken in equal quantity are mixed with loose curd. Make the mixture dry and grind it. Nila narakathin koombu, cherukadaladi koombu, chulli koombu are taken in equal quantity and grind them. Both the first and second mixture are applied to the head simultaneously.

Then Ācārya describes about the disease namely varpu which is otherwise known as **cancer** in modern medicinal system. It describes about various types of cancers namely akavarpu, puravarpu, rudira varpu, anavarpu, kuthira varpu etc. but the medicines are prescribed in common for all types of cancers.

1. After grinding thulasiyila, kalankombu and thechi veru it can be applied for the treatment of cancer.
2. Root of ekanayakam mixed up with loose curd can be applied all over the body and it is a good medication for cancer.

The Acārya says that medicines for pyoderma are also effective for cancer/varpu.

Till now we had described about some of the important illness. Now we can discuss about the medicines for some of the common diseases which are not serious.

1. *For healing wounds*: It is common that children get wounds. Application of forged and powdered kavidi with coconut milk helps to heal the wound quickly.
2. Mulla koombu and kavungin pookkula ground in equal quantity and mixed with butter is used as a medicine for wounds which is even found effective for deep wounds.

Bālagrahapīḍā: This section of Āyurveda deals with the mental health of children. Here the word *graha* is used in the sense of "something that effect from external". It is commonly found in children whose parents are living in places where lack of cleanliness and misconduct is in practice. Childrens affected by this bālagraha will cry without any reason. Skandagraha, vṛkṣagraha, Śakunigraha, pūtanā-graha are some of these bālagrahas. Treatment with reasons and *snāna bali pūjās* are the medication for this disease. Some of the normal treatments for this disease are—

1. Children having this disease are allowed to lie on the clothes and can be shown to smoke of kaduku.
2. Bathing of children using the water boiled with skin of pullukera maram and uṅgu.

Even though preparation of medicines are prescribed to save the children from this disease, more importance is given to offerings, prayers and snāna balis.

While giving instructions for these treatment procedures, Ācārya mentions the treatment for pregnancy. The health of the children has an inevitable relation with the health of the mother and because of this, treatment for pregnant women becomes necessary. In this book only general treatment for pregnancy is mentioned. Treatment for women at the early pregnancy and of post-delivery stage is mentioned in this book. Bāla-cikitsā of Āyurvedic medicinal system cares about a person's health from the time when he is an embryo in his mother's womb.

Bālacikitsā—the transcript having a prime position in Āyurveda has great traditional value, but not yet prone to scientific experimentation. Let us all hope that it will prove its signi-ficance through scientific reviews and will reach to the public as soon as possible.

Bibliography

1. Kuttikrishnan. V.M, *Aṣṭāṅgahṛdaya, Śūthrasthana*, St. Joseph press, Trivandrum.
2. Raghavan Thirumulpadu, *Aṣṭāṅgadarśanam*, Kerala Bhasha institute, Tvpm, 1998.
3. Raghavan Thirumulpadu, *Ayurvedam oru avalokanam*,

DC books, 2007.
4. Raghavan Thirumulpadu, *Ayurvedam jīvithathilue,* Nishagandhi Publications, 2002
5. Govindan Vaidyan, P.M., *Aṣṭāṅgahṛdaya,* Sūtrasthāna, Devi Book Stall, Kodungallooor.
6. Thivari, P.V., *Kaṣyapasaṃhita* or *Vridhajīvakiya,* tans., Chaukamba Viswabharati, Varanasi.
7. Krishnakulli Varrier, *History of Ayurveda,* Aryavaidyasala, Kottakkal.
8. *Encyclopedia* vol. 3, State Institute of Encyclopedia Publications.

4

Bālatantra Manuscript—A Study

R. Girija

A casual perusal of the eight sections would itself suggest how comprehensive is the science of Āyurveda. This has, long before the advent of modern medical science accomplished wonders and reached perfection in most of the branches of medicine. It is a special feature of Ayurvedic treatises that many prescriptions of medicines for various diseases are also associated with the prescriptions of certain rituals, *japas* and *pūjās*.

Śrī Kalyāṇa is the author of the *Bālatantra*, a Sanskrit manuscript, which deals with various aspects of a *roga*. The *Bālatantra* is a work comprising the prayogaśāstra and other śāstras dealing with the diseases and their remedies. It is devoted to the Vaidyaka Śāstra along with the aspects of tantras and mantras. They are described in an attractive and affiliated style.

The work begins with the traditional style of Sanskrit writers. After the invocation the author begins the work describing the *aṣṭa doṣa* of women and then the *doṣa* of puruṣa such as *raktapitta, vāta ślesma, sannipāta* and the like. Then the *devatākopana, grahadoṣa, abhicārika,* etc.

The diseases due to *vāta, pitta* and *kapha* etc. make different types of mensus. He directs medicines for each of the *rogas.* The chapters are named as paṭalas. There are fourteen paṭalas in this text. Each paṭala is devoted to a particular subject. In each paṭala various sub-subjects are dealt with. For e.g: *iti pittāhata-puṣpalakṣaṇa-cikitsā.* In the first paṭala there are fourty-six *padyas.* At the end of the first paṭala—iti *Śrīkalyāṇakṛte Bālatantre . . . vandhyāpratikāro nāma paṭalam.* In the paṭalas there are the rogavistāra, its medicines, *devatā kopa* puṣpāhatalakṣana; its *pūjās* are also dealt with.

After the mensus ladies are advised to drink the milk of cow mixed with medicines. In the second paṭala medicines are prescribed. They are *sādhāraṇa vandhyouṣadha.* The second paṭala ends with the above-said *kathana.* The third paṭala is devoted to the men having various *rogas* which make them vigourless.

In this paṭala general causes of barrenness in women and impotence in men are described and it prescribes many medicines to remove these defects. It deals with the treatment of pregnant women to safeguard the child in the womb. In this connection a description of the development of the child in every month of pregnancy is given. The causes of abortion and its treatment, diseases probable during pregnancy and medicines to cure them, necessary precautions for a safe and natural delivery—all have been described. How the mother and child are to be attended to after delivery, food of the mother and child, medicines for promoting the mother's milk—all these are dealt with in details.

In the third paṭala *puruṣavīryavṛddhikathana* is dealt. For this, many medicines are prescribed. Then the women and men are ready for reproduction. Here also medicines, *pūjās* and *bali,* etc. are observed. The fourth paṭala is described as *garbhādhānakāla rudra snānakathanam nāma.* Then the fifth paṭala deals with the *bali* and *pūjās* in each month of pregnancy along with medicines and *dānas* of various types. Thus from the very beginning of pregnancy to the last month of pregnancy are attended to in great detail.

The pregnant and pregnancy is to be guarded by various

types of medicines, mantras, tantras, pūjās and balis. The next paṭala is devoted to the act of delivery along with the house and room, prepared for the purpose. Then some of the medicines for *lepana* are mentioned. After the delivery, from the first day onward the child's care is considered most important. Along with this, medicines, *balis* and *pūjās* are also observed. The *dānas* of various kinds to the Brāhmaṇas have been advised. The child is cared properly every day, every month and every year upto the fourteenth year.

Each paṭala is meant for a particular aspect. From the first day to the fourteenth year several *rogas* will affect the child. This must be avoided and treated in the right time with right medicines, *pūjās* and *balis*. Thus also the *grahahārabali* is prescribed. Each month and each year a particular devatā will be worshipped.

Different medicines need to be given to the mother for the production of milk. Then the Dhātrī is introduced. The various *aṅgas* of the child should be kept clean. The *vāta, pitta, kapha, atisāra, hṛdroga, karṇaśūla,* etc. must be noticed and treated very well.

Then the making of Kaṣāyas, Kṛtas, lehyas and other medicines are dealt with care. Same way it deals with the making of medicines for *Jvaraharaṇopāyakathanam, atisāraharaṇam* and *ajīrṇaharaṇam.* One should keep the child from all types of *rogas. Kāsa, Śvāsa, kṛmi, pāṇḍu, svarabheda* owing to various reasons must be treated in time.

Then the *Śītaladevī stuti* is done by Lord Śiva to Skanda, i.e., śītalāṣṭakam. Then *Śītacikitsāthanam nāma* thirteenth paṭala. Netra, nāsika, karṇa, śiroroga, kīṭa vṛścikādi viṣaharaṇam and sarpādiviṣa etc. are noted. The fourteenth paṭala is dealt within this grantha in a very different style. This is written in samvat 1879 Mārgaśīrṣa māsa. This is a paper manuscript with Reg. No. 4802 and there is only one manuscript in the *Bālatrantra.* The modern medical science can empower itself on this subject with the help of the manuscript.

5

A Critical Study of Agastya—Yogasāram Kiḷippaṭṭu

LALU S. KURUP

Kiḷippaṭṭu is one of the wealthy traditional style of writing in Malayalam literature. By adopting this style of writing from sixteenth to twentieth century AD, about 200 literary works were composed. The Purāṇas and Epics were the central theme of these writings. The Kiḷippaṭṭu style is also used in other works covering the topics of medicine, history, etc. The work *Agastyayogasāram Kiḷippaṭṭu* belong to this category. The theme of this poem is the preparation and the usage of Siddha medicine.

Siddha is a form of South Indian Tamil traditional medicine and part of the trio-Indian Medicine—Āyurveda, Siddha and Yunani. This is nearly 10,000 years old medical system followed by the Tamil people both in India and abroad. This system of medicine was popular in ancient India due to the antiquity of the medical system.

Siddha system is believed to have been developed by the eighteen siddha in the South called 'Siddhar'.[1] They are the ancient super-natural spiritual saints of India and the Siddha system is believed to have been handed over to the Siddhars by the Hindu God Śiva and Goddess Pārvatī. They are Tirumular, Ramadevar, Agastyar, Konganavar, Kamalamuni, Chattai-muni, Karuvurar, Sundaranandar, Valmiki, Nandhidever, Pambatti, Bhokanathar, Machamuni,

Korakkar, Patañjali, Dhanwantari, Kadambai and Idaikkadar.

The Saint Agastya wrote a lot of works related to Siddha Medicine in Tamil. Some important works are Agathiar 21000, Agathiar Paripuranam, Agathiar Nayanavidhi, Agathiar Gunapadam, Agathiar Pillaitamil etc. The 'Agastya yogasāram Kilippaṭṭu' narrate the medicine 'Narasiṅghāmṛtam' which Agastyar mentioned in his works. A transcript of this work is preserved in the Oriental Research Institute and Manuscripts Library of the Kerala University (T.No. 987). It is an anonymous work having 188 lines. This describes various diseases of human beings and its treatments including remedies. It is an unpublished work. Therefore its study is more significant.

The work begins with a note on the ingredients of the medicine, its quantity and the various methods applied for its purification. Then the work sheds light on the usage and benefits of Narasiṁghāmṛtam. The work ends with different types of diseases which affect mankind and how they are treated with the use of Narasiṁghāmṛta sevā. Though there is no evidence about the author, the study focuses on its medicinal importance.

Contents

In Siddha there were 64 types of medicines for both internal and external use

- *Internal medicine* was used through the oral route and further classified into 32 categories based on their form, methods of preparation, shelf life, etc.
- *External medicine* includes certain forms of drugs and also certain applications like nasal, eye and ear drops and also certain procedures like leech application. It is also classified into thirty-two categories.

These medicines are prepared from plants (herbal product), dhātu (inorganic substances), jaṅgama (animal products), natural plants, minerals, (lavanagal), the inner parts of living organisms, etc.

In this work, the method of making Narasiṁghāmṛtam is described from line number 16 to 25. Asparagus, Sugar, Ghee, Honey, Gingelly seed, Thina seed, Herddaturased were the ingredients of the Lehyam. The usage of Narasiṁghāmṛtam is explained in line 30 and 31 of this work. In these lines the dosage and time for taking medicine is also mentioned.

Pathyas

The success of Siddha medicine depends on *pathya*, which is essentially a list of do's and don'ts. The patient should follow *pathya* for keeping the quality of medicine beneficial in order to cure his/her illness. Siddha medicine is claimed to revitalize and rejuvenate dysfunctional organs that cause the disease and to maintain the balance of *vāta, pitta* and *kapha*. In Siddha medicine system, diet and lifestyle play a major role not only in health but also for curing diseases. But there is no *pathya* or conditions to be followed after taking the dose of Narasiṁghāmṣtam. But the mind of the patient needs to be pure and peaceful for achieving good results.

The work claimes that Narasiṁghāmṛtam is very effective and it was used as a medicine for all diseases like Leprosy, Syphilis, Crysipelas and also one can apply it for headache.

Conclusion

Siddha medicine is an amulgam of Science, Medicine, Spirituality and Philosophy. Here, importance is given to the patient and not to his/her disease. So while conducting the treatment physical condition of the patient is also taken into consideration. The Siddha medicine got wide popularity because it can cure the most complicated illness without any side effects. Likewise the ability to recover health and smartness to both men and women, with the help of Narasiṁghāmṛtam gained support from people. It is very clear that the kilipattu style of literature can be taken into the traditional medical fields.

Note

1. The Tamil work named 'Maruthuva Vathayoga Jñāna Śāstram' gives more details about the 18 Siddhars.

Bibliography

1. Agastya Yogasaram Kilippattu (Transcript copy number 987), Thiruvananthapuram: Oriental Research Institute and Manuscripts Library.
2. Anaivāri R. Anandan (Editor) A Compendium of Siddha Doctrine, Chennai: Dept. of Indian Medicine and Homoeopathy, 2005.
3. Sambasivam Pillai, T.V., Introduction to Siddha Medicine, Madras: Dept. of Indian Medicine and Homoeopathy, 1993.
4. Sambasivam Pillai, T.V., Tamil—English Dictionary vol. IV, Chennai Dept. of Indian Medicine and Homoeopathy, 1998.
5. Shanmugavelan A, Siddhar's Science of Longevity and Kalpa Medicine of India, Madras, Directorate of Dept. of Indian Medicine and Homoeopathy, 1992.

6

Interpretation, Adaptation and Translation—Process of Pratisaṃskaraṇa

K. MUTHULEKSHMI

One important characteristic of intellectual discourses in Sanskrit is the importance given to the 'text'. Each discipline considers some texts to be its foundation. Sūtra texts of different systems of philosophy are examples. The recognition of Śruti as *pramāṇa* also points to this infallible authority ascribed to text. In Āyurveda, texts like the *Carakasaṃhitā*, the *Suśruta-saṃhitā* and the *Aṣṭāngahṛdaya* together are considered to be *Bṛhattrayī* (three major texts) of the Śāstra. Even the gradual steps of the learning process were also designed as a process that progresses from one text to another. So, there is enough space for making out a 'text science' related to intellectual discourses in Sanskrit.

Such importance ascribed to the texts of course reflects a sense of continuity through ages. No knowledge system can persist unless it addresses the contemporary issues and problems. For this purpose, the fundamental texts were renewed and reconstructed time and again. One of the ways through which this was accomplished was through different commentaries written on the text. These commentaries served different functions, which included making the text capable of addressing contemporary issues. It can be said that such hermeneutic engagements were always inherent to Sanskrit tradition.

Text–Formation and Interpretation.

Since texts were regarded as authoritative in a system of thought, specific rules were laid down for the formation of texts. Actually, 'text' is not just the ideas contained in it. But there are many factors which determine it. The frame of *anubandhacatuṣṭaya* is one of them. The four *anubandha*-s are *adhikārī, viṣaya, sambandha* and *prayojana*. Each one of these components is important in its own way. They are indicative of the persons the text addresses (*adhikārī*), the subject matter discussed (*viṣaya*), relation between the text and subject matter or between reader and the speaker (*sambandha*) and the effect that the text makes upon the reader (*prayojana*). It is through these four components that the text relates to the outer world. It is also how the outer world determines the text. These factors fix or specify the place of the text against a broad background of ideas. The reader of the text, his/her responses to the text, the effect the text makes on the reader—all these are to be taken into consideration for assuming what a text is. For example, one of the introductory verses in the Aṣṭāṅgahṛdaya is the following.

āyuḥ kāmayamānena
dharmārthasukhasādhanam/
āyrvedopadeśeṣu
vidheyaḥ paramādaraḥ.[1]

(One who is desirous of obtaining *āyuḥ* which is the tool for *dharma, artha* and *sukha,* he/she should show supreme respect for suggestions of Āyurveda.)

This verse has been interpreted as pointing to the *anubandhacatuṣṭaya* of Āyurveda. One who is desirous of attaining *āyuḥ* is *adhikārī* here. *Āyurvedopadeśa*-s are the *viṣaya*-s, *ādaraḥ* (respect) is *sambandha* and *āyuḥ* which gives *dharma, artha* and *sukha* is *prayojanam*. Such a preconception about the text makes the communication easier and clear.

Another text-forming method relevant in this regard is the *adhikaraṇa* method. An *adhikaraṇa* is a self-contained unit, comprising of the six elements of *viṣaya, saṃśaya, pūrvapakṣa, uttara, saṅgati* and *phala*. The subject-matter, through *adhikaraṇa* method, gets a systematic way of expression. And the subject-matter could be presented against the background of different perspectives (*saṃśaya* and *pūrvapakṣa*). Even though each *adhikaraṇa* is a self- contained unit, they are linked together as a text by the element of *saṅgati*. Saṅgati is the specific order in which different *adhikaraṇa*-s are arranged in a text. The order of topics is much relevant in representing the general outlook of the text. Many examples can be pointed out with regard to this from the texts of Sanskrit philosophical literature. This is also evident from the way adaptations are made out of texts.

Both these methods of *anubandhacatuṣṭaya* and *adhikaraṇalakṣaṇa* can be used as tools for studying about interpretations, adaptations and translations of books of different disciplines. Even though these rules seem to limit or fix the space of a text to a certain measure, it can be seen that a subtle shift in these could make the text anew.

Pratisaṃskaraṇam

Ayurvedic way of making the text contemporary is termed *pratisaṃskaraṇa*. Āyurveda-ācārya-s have always acknowledged the need of making the text compatible with the changing times. Vāgbhaṭa says—

svānyatantravirodhanam
    bhuyiṣṭham vinivārakaḥ
yugānurupasandarbho
    vibhāgena kariṣyate[2]

(Having solved the contradictions in one's own and also

other Śāstra-s, this text is being made contemporary, through restructuring the order of topics.)

This verse indicates both the mechanism and functions of making the text *yugānurūpasandarbha*.
Following verse by Caraka also emphasizes this point.

"*Agniveśakṛte tantre Carakapratisaṃskṛte*"[3]
(In this Śāstra made by Agniveśa, which has been *pratisaṃskṛta* by Caraka.

It is known from *vyākhyāna*-s that it was Nāgārjuna who made the text *Suśrutasaṃhitā pratisaṃskṛta.*

saṃskartā kurute tantram
purāṇaṃ ca punarnavam[4]
(One who makes the text *saṃskṛta*, makes the old text renewed—*Suśrutasaṃhitā.*)

The process of *pratisaṃskaraṇa* was made possible through conscious efforts of textual reconstruction. As the basic texts of many reconstructed texts have become extant now, we cannot directly analyse the ways of this process.

Modern adaptations and translations
By about 16th/17th centuries, a basic shift was evident in intellectual discourses. In the place of traditional forms of interpretation, adaptations and translations to different languages were brought out. These were not just a technical processes of change in language, but one that had great cultural, social and intellectual impact. Analysing the mechanism of modern adaptations and translations employing the traditional methodologies of *anubandhacatuṣṭaya* and *adhikaraṇasvarūpa* will be interesting.
Important modern day adaptations of the basic Āyurvedic texts of the *Carakasaṃhitā*, the *Suśrutasaṃhitā* and *Aṣṭāṅ-*

gahṛdaya are the legacy of Caraka, the legacy of Suśruta and the legacy of Vāgbhaṭa written by Dr.M.S.Valiathan. These adaptations address the modern day readers (a different kind of *adhikārī*) in a different context. The relation between the text and the reader has also undergone a change from that of the age of *Carakasaṃhitā*. These changes surely bring out a new *prayojana* upon the reader. Thus the *viṣaya* itself becomes a new one. Thus the newly formed *anubandha-catuṣṭaya* places the new text in a new plane.

For analysing the mechanism of adaptation adopted by Dr. M.S. Valiathan, the *adhikaraṇa* method can be applied. The element of *saṅgati* of *adhikaraṇa* is more relevant in this regard. As mentioned earlier, *saṅgati* is the order of topics in the whole text. The structure of the text reflects the outlook of the text in general. Vāgbhaṭa has reminded about the importance of *saṅgati* thus—

> "*te'rthāḥ sa granthabandhaśca*
> *saṃkṣepāya kramo'nyathā.*[5]
> (The very same ideas, the very same structure,but another order has been followed for conveying the ideas briefly.)

Here the emphasis is upon abridging the ideas. But another order can be followed for other purposes. The general order and division of topics in the *Carakasaṃhitā* etc. are in the following manner:

1. Sūtrasthāna—basic principles
2. Śarīrasthāna—physiology and anatomy
3. Nidānasthāna—pathology
4. Cikitsāsthāna—stages of disease, methods of treatment
5. Kalpasthāna—manufacturing, collection etc. of medicines.
6. Uttarasthāna—portions other than kāyacikitsā
7. Vimānasthāna—methods of teaching, learning and discussion.

8. Siddhisthāna—fruits of treatment

A modern day reader might be confused to find that the details relating to a single disease are scattered in different chapters of the text. The logic behind this kind of division of topics is the holistic vision the Ācārya-s had maintained. Health was not viewed from the point of view of disease or treatment. It was viewed as a positive state of equilibrium of body, mind and surroundings.

For the modern day reader, this kind of holistic approach may seem unpractical. Today, health is viewed from the point of view of disease and treatment. So for communicating with the modern day readers, Dr. Valiathan has restructured the whole text accordingly. After the introductory portions dealing with fundamental principles, he arranges chapters on the basis of disease and treatment. He has codified the details of each disease chapterwise. This enables the reader to get all the details of each disease from one portion of text itself. Here it is evident that two different orders of arrangement of topics refer to two different approaches to the subject. While the modern reader views health from the point of disease and treatment, Āyurveda Śāstra views it from the point of a positive state of life, which is beyond the realm of medicines and treatment.

Dynamics of translation

As the adaptations of Dr.Valiathan are in English language, they can be considered to be translations also. The shift from Sanskrit language to English language has made a great difference. These reconstructed texts have readers at a global level and they evoke global level responses too.

The translation of these texts into Malayalam evokes regional level responses and discussions. The change in language makes a new set of *anubandhacatuṣṭaya* which acts as the vehicle of cultural and intellectual transactions.

Each language constitutes a different *anubandhacatuṣṭaya*

and and each of them functions as complimentary to each other.

Continuity/discontinuity

The long and varied history of evolution of ancient Śāstra-s undergoes phases of both continuity and discontinuity. Both phases are important in their own way. Continuity is important in the sense that each Śāstra maintains its own indigenous character. It has to be understood from that perspective. Discontinuity is important in the sense that new knowledge in the field has to be incorporated to the old stock, some notions reviewed and reconstructed. The underlying mechanism that operates behind these aspects of continuity and discontinuity is very much relevant in understanding their course of evolution. Modern methodologies are widely used for such studies nowadays. Here, an attempt is made to examine the aspects of continuity and discontinuity with regard to the discipline of Āyurveda using traditional methodological tools.

References

1. *Aṣṭāṅgahṛdayam,* 1.2; Śārārthabodhinī commentary by Poyya Raman Menon. Published by V.K.R T. Foundation, Chalakudy, 2010.
2. *Aṣṭāṅgahṛdayam,* 1.20.
3. Colophone in each chapter of *Carakasaṃhitā*
4. *Carakasaṃhitā,* Siddhisthānam, 12.36
5. *Aṣṭāṅgahṛdayam,* 1.22.

7

Vaidyaka Manuscripts in the Oriental Research Institute and Manuscripts Library, Thiruvananthapuram

P.L. SHAJI

The department of Oriental Research Institute and Manuscripts Library of the University of Kerala has got the largest palmleaf manuscript collection in India, where almost 65,000 works can be found preserved in around 30,000 bundles, 80% of which are palm-leaves. It can very well be noticed that there is no subject which our ancestors left out. Less than 2% of the manuscripts are dated ones and 150-600 years old.

There are 3700 Vaidya Granthas and the languages in which are been written are Sanskrit, Tamil, Malayalam, Hindi, Marathi, etc. and the scripts vary from Devanagari, Malayalam, Tamil, to even Marathi. Most of the Sanskrit works have interpretations in both Malayalam and Sanskrit. Different forms of literature like Manipravālam and Kilipattu style could also be seen. Most of the Vaidya Grandhas are seen to be written in poetic form like other works of science and literature.

Many forms of science existed for the betterment of mankind and they were and are still useful. "The experiments and studies conducted in the foremost life science branches like molecular biology reveal that our ancient codified knowledge and scientific knowledge hold good to a limit of 100%.

Our traditional indigenous medicines have evolved from the experiences that were collected from the surroundings through ages. Those who want to study the system of medicines (indigenous) of Kerala will have to go deep into the manuscripts of those times.

Our ancestors found out cure for common ailments from the clements available in the surroundings. These types of traditional medicines was noted in the drawings in caves, then in palm leaves and afterwards in handmade paper. They wrote it down for the use of the generations to come.

When Āyurveda is being discussed here, it is important to consider that some *granthas* prevailed even before Āyurveda came into existence. There is a mention of Āyurveda in the *Atharvaveda*, the *Taittārīyaponiṣad* and the *Garbhopaniṣad.* Similarly, we get some indications of the indigenous medicines in the *Agnipurāṇa* and in some Tantra manuscripts.

The three pillars of Āyurveda are Caraka, Suśruta and Vāgbhaṭa. The Carakasaṃhitā system of treatment has been divided into three. The system of treatment involving enchantment in Mantra and Tantra is called *daivavya-pāśrayam.* That involving yoga and meditations is called *satvāśrayam.* The third one is *yuktyupāśrayam,* which is based on the five elements of matter as all living beings are made of *pañcabhūtas.*

In earlier times Sanskrit Vaidya granthas gained popularity.The Vaidya granthas of Caraka and Suśruta, prevailed in Kerala. But later the system of Buddhist disciple Vāgbhaṭa, namely *Aṣṭāṅgasaṅgraha* and *Aṣṭāṅgahṛdaya* gained popularity. Different interpretations written in different periods could be found in the libraries.

The *Yogasāra* and the *Mahāsāra* combined mantra, yantra and medicines. The *granthas* prove that such systems were common those days. Even now there is a system of visiting priests, mantrics and sannyāsis for the cure of ailments.

The indigenous/traditional medicine system of Kerala

includes Marma cikitsā, Bāla cikitsā, Netra cikitsā, Viṣa cikitsā (Toxicology). Post-delivery care, etc. Medicines have been prescribed for fracture as well.

There is only one incomplete copy for the *Rasavaiśeṣikasūtra* viz. *Vaidyamanoramā* a grantha with Malayalam notes which deals with antidotes. The independent work of Śrī. Pullanthol Moosathu named Cikitsāmañjarī, contains indigenous *rogas* and treatment plans. Copies of the text are available in the department.

The *Rasamañjarī* of 'Vaidyanatha Suda Saleenatha explains how to make *rasa bhasma* and it has been explained as a medicine for maintaining youth if consumed in the proper way. Sulphur (*gandhaka*) has been explained as a medicine and procedure for obtaining pure fresh sulphur has also been mentioned in the text.

There are nine *granthas* which deal with pregnancy and its care. These works are about customary style of pregnancy care.

The manuscripts in the library deal with the treatment of human beings, and animals as well. There is a mention of veterinary science. Pālakapya, Mātaṅgalīlā, Gajacikitsā, Aśvacikitśa, etc. deal with the common diseases of elephants, horses etc. which proves that there were treatment for animals also. There are six interpretations and four Manipravala kṛtis for *Mātaṅgalīlā*. Marma treatment is another important aspect of Āyurveda. There are many works on this subject in Sanskrit, Malayalam and Tamil. It deals with cardinal points of the body, the ailments that can come on these cardinal points and their treatment. There are fifty-one works on Marma Śāstra. They are *marmacikitsā*, Marmalakṣaṇam kiṭipattu, Marmalakṣaṇavum and cikitsāsavum, Marmavijñānam, Marmabhikatheśaṃhithā, etc. There are some Marma treatment *granthas* for elephants, namely Mātaṅgamarma, Gajamarmacikitsā, etc.

The division of Toxicology has 122 Malayalam *granthas*. *Viṣacandrikā, Viṣacikitsā, Viśanārāyanīyam, Viṣanāśanam,*

Viṣaharamantram, Viṣaharaṇam trangals deal with the treatment for the poison of snakes, lizards etc. The Dūtalakṣaṇam deals with the subject whether a person who has been bitten by snake will survive or not.

The eight major branches of Āyurveda are *Śalya* (Surgery), *Sālākya* (eyes, ears etc.), *Kāyacikitsā* (whole body), *Bhūtavidyā* (psychotherapy) *Kaumārabhṛtya* the pediatrics) *Agadatantra* (antidotes), *Rasāyanatantra* (preparation and application of elixirs), *Vijikaraṇatantra* (aphrodisiacs), etc.

Śalya-cikitsā gives importance to surgery and four *granthas* are available on this subject. Suśruta manuscripts deal with *Śalya-cikitsā.* There are no separate manuscript for Śālākya cikitsā, *Vājikaraṇatantra, Rasāyana-cikitsā,* etc. They are dealt in common *granthas* for treatment. There are separate manuscripts for ophthalmic treatment. There are eight *granthas* for ophthalmology of which two are complete.

Āyurveda will become complete only when the Caraka-Suśruta *granthas* which follow Sanskrit tradition are assimilated to this system. The manuscript *Nirantara padavyākhyā* is a commentary on *Carakasaṃhitā* which is commandable even though it is incomplete and has not been published yet.

The *Aṣṭāṅgahṛdaya,* written by Vāgbhaṭa, a Buddhist is the quintessence of the works of Caraka and Suśruta (6th AD) even though it is an independent work. Kerala tradition follows the *Aṣṭāṅgahṛdaya* and the *Aṣṭāṅgasaṅgraha.* There are many commentaries in Sanskrit and in Malayalam which were very popular in Kerala.

The *Yogāmṛtam,* the *Yogasāram, Cikitsāmañjarī* etc. have been published. Śrī Uppottukannan, wrote the first interpretation to the *Aṣṭāṅgahṛdaya.* The *Cikitsāmañjarī* is an old *grantha,* but many portions are same as in *Yogāmṛtam.* Hence it can be concluded that the *Cikitāsmañjarī* was written after the *Yogāmṛtam.* In the copies, it could very well be seen that the Vaidyas of those times, when copied/ and printed the text, added their views on treatments from their own experience.

The *Bhelasaṃhitā* of Bhelācārya was written in second century. This department has an incomplete copy of the same. He had said that the portion of mind is in the brain and that a type of juice which emanates from the heart circulates all over the body and comes back to the heart. This was written centuries before William Harvy found out circulation of blood.

There are medical dictionaries also which enrich the collection of the Oriental Research Institute. They include *Madanādi nighaṇṭu, Auṣadhinighaṇṭu Rasanighaṇṭu, Rājanigāṇḍu* and *Vaidyanighaṇṭu* etc. The Madanādinighaṇṭu was published by this Department in 2005.

Conclusion

From all the above descriptions, it could be very well be assessed, how rich and varied the traditional medicine system was. There is no such disease which has not been mentioned for its cure. How rich the awareness of our Ācāryas would have been. It had cure for terminal diseases also even before the discovery of modern medicines. It identified the principles like circulation of blood, importance of our brain and heart, cardinal points of the body, etc.

It may be noted that often this indigenous system of medicine had combined the aspects of Mantra and Tantra, in order to give motivation to the patient and thereby obtaining positive results. Āyurveda prescribes veterinary medicines also. From the medical dictionaries it is revealed that almost all the flora and fauna has medical effects and their easy availability had given impetus to the preparation and practice of Āyurveda/Vaidya in this part of the country. Even now it can be concluded that Vaidya tradition is retained in Kerala without tampering its traditional purity and quality.

References

1. *Alphbetical Index of Sanskrit Manuscripts in the Oriental Research Institute and Manuscripts Library*, University of Kerala, Trivandrum, Volume 1 to 7, 1957–88
2. Index of Malayalam Manuscripts, Subject-wise. Oriental Research Institute and Manuscripts Library, University of Kerala, Trivandrum, 1996
3. *Technical Literature in Sanskrit,* ed., Dr. S. Venkitasubramonia Iyer, Department of Publication, University of Kerala, Trivandrum, 1978.

8

Ayurveda—A Vibrant Tradition of Kerala

K.G. Sreelekha

Āyurveda is India's traditional and natural system of medicine that has been practised for more than five thousand years. It is one of India's great gifts to the mankind. The term 'āyus' means duration or span of life and the term 'veda' means unimpeachable knowledge. So it is commonly translated as the science of life or is the science of living in harmony with nature. It is a holistic system that gives man proper guidelines for a full and balanced life by establishing a state of harmony and inner peace that is necessary for our integral well being. It advises a proper code of living with guidelines for diet, sleep, meditation, mantra and prayer, massage and oil baths, the use of herbs and yoga practice.

The history of Āyurveda starts from the time of the Vedas. They preach the philosophy of life. The *Atharvaveda* contains the principles of healing on which Āyurveda is based. It has influenced many of the older traditional methods of healing including Tibetan, Chinese, and Greek medicine. Āyurveda is considered by many as the 'mother of healing'. It is the system of health care conceived and developed by the *ṛṣis* and natural scientists through centuries of observations, experiments, discussions and meditations. For several thousand years their teachings were passed orally from teacher to student.

Āyurveda emphasizes prevention of diseases, rejuvenation

of our body systems and extension of life span. The profound premise and promise of Āyurveda tell us that through certain practices, not only can we prevent heart disease and make our headaches go away we can but better understand ourselves and the world around us, live a long healthy life in balance and harmony, achieve our fullest potential and express our true inner nature on a daily basis.

According to Āyurveda every human being is a creation of the cosmos, the pure cosmo consciousness of two energies—male energy called Puruṣa and female energy, Prakṛti. Puruṣa is choiceless passive awareness, while Prakṛti is choiceful active energy.

Āyurveda provides an integrated approach to preventing and treating illness through lifestyle interventions and natural therapies. It is based on the view that the element forces and principles that comprise all of nature and that holds it together and make it function are also seen in human beings. In Āyurveda the mind and the body not only influence each other, they are part of each other. Together they form the mind-body. Ayurvedic philosophy and practices link us to every aspect of ourselves and remind us that we are in union with every aspect of nature, as well as the entire universe.

There cannot be good mental health without good physical health and vice versa. In Āyurveda symptoms of diseases that could be catagorised as mental thoughts or feelings are important elements for diseases of the physical body. Both are due to imbalances within a person and both are treated by restoring the natural balance mentally and physically. In Āyurveda your whole life and lifestyle must be in harmony before you can enjoy true well being. Life style interventions are a major Ayurvedic preventive and therapeutic approach.

The ideal geographic location of Kerala and its climate has made external purification and rejuvenation therapies most effective for treatment of many psychosomatic disorders. The high humidity in Kerala helps to open up the body pores and the medicinal oils used in massaging get easily absorbed in the body by increasing the effectiveness of the treatment.

The fundamentals of Āyurveda being practised and taught in Kerala are not different from those of the rest of the country in their essence and philosophy. But in the present days there indeed is a notable difference in certain aspects of Kerala tradition of Āyurveda. This difference pertains to the importance given to Vāgbhaṭa's *Aṣṭāṅgahṛdaya* in preference to other classical texts by Kerala traditional physicians.

Kerala is proud of the traditional system of medical treatment called Āyurveda. From very ancient times Ayurvedic treatment was very popular in Kerala. Kerala made rich contributions to the theory and practice of the medical science by its active research in improving the traditional system.

The development of Āyurveda in Kerala is particularly noted in non-brahmanical traditions even before the entry of classical Āyurveda in the early centuries of the Christian era. These two streams subsequently blended so well that it gave an unique strength to the health care tradition of Kerala. Selected few Brahmin households named generally as Aṣṭavaidyas were bestowed with the responsibility of maintaining the Ayurvedic tradition by practicing it as a health care service as well as by teaching its principles in the unique gurukula tradition. The traditional practitioners of Āyurveda considered Aṣṭāṅgahṛdaya as a primary text. Several commentaries of this text were written by experts both in Malayalam and Sanskrit. The *Sahasrayogam,* the *Cikitsāmañjarī,* the *Vaidyamanoramā* are just few examples. These and similar other Kerala texts still remain sources of very useful informations on formulation of medicinal plants and therapies.

It is believed that Vāgbhaṭa the author of the Ayurvedic grantha, *Aṣṭāṅgahṛdaya* and *Aṣṭṅgasaṅgraha* wrote them when he was staying in Kerala and his disciples popularized this system of treatment. It was the Buddhists who gave extensive popularity to the Ayurvedic system of medicine in Kerala. The Buddhist monasteries had dispensaries which supplied medicines to the sick people and provided medical aid to animals also. The temples in Kerala gave medical preparations or oils to mentally and physically sick devotees and thus played an important role in the popularizaiton of Ayurvedic treatment.

The original and authentic books on Āyurveda were written in Sanskrit. There are a number of works in Malayalam describing the Āyurveda system of medicine and *Sarvāṅgacikitsāratnam, Vaidyamanoramā, Vaidyamañjarī,* etc. are the most important among them. There were plenty of works on special branches like Toxicology, Paediatrics, Gynecology, Opthalmology and diseases like Leprosy, Diabetes, Tuberculosis, Rheumatism, etc.

The impact of Āyurveda is deep-rooted in Kerala society. This system got acceptance and popularity in this region from very early period. There exist traditional families who engage themselves in the practice of Āyurveda. Such families can be seen without having any caste or religious restriction.

Important works on Āyurveda were well studied and exhaustive commentaries on them were produced by Keralites. Among the Ayurvedic works, Vāgbhaṭa's *Aṣṭāṅga-hṛdaya* is the most popular one in Kerala. Several commentaries of this work are found in this region. Among them Vākyapradīpikā of Alattur Prakeswaran Nambi, Kairalai commentary by Planthol Moosad, Aṣṭāṅgahṛdayavyākhyā of Govinda Pisharadi are a few examples. The Aṣṭāṅgahṛdaya-koṣa of K.M.Vaidyar provides the technical terms of text arranged in alphabetical order. There are many independent works and commentaries by Kerala authors. The *Viṣanārāyaṇīyam* of Nārāyaṇa, a sixteenth century work on toxicology, is an authoritative one. Hṛdayapriyā of Vaikkathu Paccummoothatu is a major work and it contains four parts consisting of sixty chapters. This popular work is of 1865 and published under Trivandrum Sanskrit Series (TSS 111). The *Sukhasādhaka* is an abridgement of *Hṛdayapriya.* It is written by the same author and is of 1881. Vadakkeppat Narayan Nair brought out *Anugraha-mīmaṃsā* in six sections. This work deals with Bacteriology. It incorporates some western ideas also. Another work *Bṛhatśarīrika* in 21 chapters by the same author deals with human Anatomy and Physiology combining Indian and Western systems. The *Sadācāravṛttivardhana* a work of Āryasarman consists of 17 chapters. It discusses both Vaidya, and Vedānta. *Sarvagaralapramocana* of Kuttamath Rama Kurup is a valuable work having 12 chapters. This work deals with the treatment of poison. The *Yogasārasaṃgraha* of Vasudeva explains different kinds of medicinal preparations. *Ārogayśāstra* of Kudungalloor Kochunni Thampuran with his own commentary is a noteworthy publication. The *Rasatantra* of A.R. Rajarajavarma and the *Rasamañjarī* of Thaikkat Narayan Moosad deal with Rasāyanatrantra. Cikitsāsthāna of Keralavarma Ilayaraja of Cochin Palace, *Hṛdayollāsa* commentary of the *Suśrutasaṃhitā* by Vasudeva Sarma and his Malayalam commentaries for *Carakasaṃhitā. Sukhasādhaka, Aṣṭasthānaprakāśikā* and *Yogaratnākara* require special mention. K.M. Narayanam Vaidyar's Malayalam commentaries on the *Suśrutasaṃhitā* and Sūtrasthāna of *Aṣṭāṅgahṛdaya* are very valuable. The commentary of the *Carakasaṃhitā* by T.C. Parameswaran Moosad, the commentary on *Aṣṭāṅgahṛdaya* by Vasudevan Moosad, the Malayalam commentary 'Prakāśikā' *Aṣṭāṅgahṛdaya* by Raghavan Tirumulpad, Sārārthadarpaṇa commentary on *Aṣṭaṅgahṛdaya* by Kaikulangara Rama Variyar, Aruṇodaya commentary on the *Aṣṭāṅgahṛdaya* by Kayikkara Govindan Vaidyar, the Gūḍhārthacandrikā commentary by Cheppatt Acuta Variyar, Sārabodhinī commentary on *Aṣṭāṅgahṛdaya* by Kochusankaran Vaidyan, a Malayalam commentary on the same text by Sreekanta are some valuable commentaries on

Ayurvedic *granthas* by Kerala authors. In addition to this, many commentaries on the *Aṣṭāṅgahṛdaya* in different languages are popular in Kerala. A few among them are Nidānacintāmaṇi, Bālabodhini, Hṛdya, Lalitā and Saṅketamañjarī.

The *Sūtikāmṛtam* written by Kayikkara Govindan Vaidyar is a commendable publication. His translation of *Aṣṭāṅgahṛdaya* entitled *Aṣṭāṅgahṛdayabhāṣā* is a work to be specially mentioned. So also the Malayalam translation of the same text by Kesavan Embranthiri is a useful contribution to this field. There is a Maṇipravālakāvya in Āyurveda and its name is *Yogāmṛta.*

Prayogasamuccaya written by Kerala Varma of Cochin is considered to be an authoritative work on toxicology. Kerala also contributed popular Ayurvedic dictionaries like *Āyurveda Nighaṇṭu* and *Āyurveda Ratnākarakoṣam. Śarīram* and *Ārogyamārgaṅgal* of Dr.L.A. Ravivarma also enriched the Ayurvedic literature. Dr. P.S. Warrier's *Aṣṭāṅgaśarīra* and *Bṛhaccharīra* are also notable contributions to Āyurveda.

Āyurveda literature was enriched by other scholars also. Pachumoothathu the author of *Thiruvithamkoor Charitam* was an expert physician. He wrote two medical books *Hṛdayapriyā* and *Sukhasādhakam.* Mahakavi Vallathol contributed *Ārogyacintāmaṇi, Garbharakṣākramam* and *Vaidyajīvanam.*

In the methods of treatment also Kerala has an unique tradition. The *pañcakarma* treatment had been resorted by the Ayurvedic physicians of Kerala from very early days. Dhara, Njavarakizhi, Pizhichil, Uzhichil, etc. are reckoned as special treatments of Kerala. The *Dhārākalpam* deals with the Dhārā treatment. *Vaidyamanoramā* contains numerous clinical applications. There are also a number of books dealing with treatment such as *Sahasrayogam, Cikitsākramam, Vaidyamañjarī, Cikitsāmañjari, Yogāmṛtam, Sannipātacikitsā, Netrarogacikitsā, Masūrimalacikitsā,* etc. *Mātaṅgalīlā* deals with the treatment of elephants.

Kerala has a number of special medicinal herbs and plants.

There are fifty dictionaries of these medicinal plants and herbs. During the Dutch period Henry Van Rheede, the Dutch Governor in Kerala took interest in the compilation of a dictionary describing the medicinal properties of Indian plants. The result was the compilation of *Hortus Malabaricus* in twelve volumes.

The practice of Āyurveda treatment was the chief occupation of a number of families from the time of the Sangam Age or even prior to that period. There are references of the Velavaidyas in the Sangam works. Physicians in Āyurveda sprang up form different communities like the Ezhavas, Ganakas, Mannans, Brahmins, Nairs and among the Christians also arose great physicians. The Aṣṭavaidyas of Kerala are very famous. They belong to eight Brahmin families and they claim that they were the disciples of Vāgbhaṭa who was the great authority on Āyurveda.

Āyurveda in Kerala has a particular place than all other Āyurveda destinations all over the world. People from different parts of India as well as from foreign countries flock to Kerala Ayurvedic treatment centres to experience the virtues of the best Āyurveda health packages. What makes Kerala Āyurveda tradition unique is the special interest people here have been taking for centuries to foster Āyurveda in many ways. As a result, Āyurveda in Kerala has crossed the boundary of being a mere herbal healing system and grown into a place of interest to the researchers.

9

Nayanavithi Vākatam

Kum. Radha

Introduction

Sweet Tamil, I live of thee
Want not even the ambrosia of Gods

So say the scholars who enjoy and experience the penacea of Tamil language. Tamil is known for its reputed ancient heritage as well as modern greatness. It is rich in having a large number of books on various subjects such as Literature, Grammar, Drama, Music, Medicine and Prophecy. These treasures of books were transcribed and preserved in the form of palm-leaf manuscripts. Most of the books so far published are based on these manuscripts. Among the manuscripts available today mostly are medical manuscripts. They offer the guidelines too.

Those who are wise to foresee the pain of evil
guard themselves against surprise shocks. (*Thirukkural* 429)

According to the words of Thiruvalluvar one can help himself to prevent diseases before their entry.

The Tamil word *noi* (disease) derives from the base word *no* which means pain or suffering. Disease is the one which blocks the normal activities of the physical organs and instigates suffering in the body. If a person is affected by a disease, his normal skills will become null, however healthy he be. In that critical situation, he who cures the disease is considered to be the life-giver. This is known by the proverb:

Physician is like father
All inhabitants are his friends.

Even the classical work *Tholkappiam* points out:

Paiyal and lowliness are the
meanings of disease.

Disease is common and unavoidable in everyone's life. Knowing the nature of diseases, men of early times discovered medicine and followed specific methods of treatment. It spreads its branches widely as Allopathy, Homoeopathy, Unani, Ayurvedic, Acupuncture and Siddha medicine.

Among the above-mentioned treatments, the most-used Tamil medicine is today's 'Siddha medicine'. It is said that the Siddhars found this method of treatment based on the prophecy of the Lord Śiva. It is said in the Northern Legends that Lord Śiva granted Northern Language to Pāṇini and Tamil to Agathiyar. There is a proof from an old song:

Āthiyil Tamil nool Agathiyarukku
Unarththiya Māthorupāhan.

(Initially, the Lord who is the half of a woman gave Tamil book to Agathiyar). So it is believed that the Siddhars followed the sage Agathiyar and from him they learnt and brought out the Siddha medicine to the world.

As the head is the greatest part of human body, so is the 'eye' among the senses. Whenever the body is affected with any disease, the Siddhars follow the treatment carefully.

They found rare treatment methods to treat the softest organ of the body 'eye'. They have some classifications to find out the nature of a normal healthy eye; the changes in the eye when it is affected; diagnosing the disease based on the symptoms; prescribing suitable medicines, methods of preparation, dosage of medicines, diseases which can be cured with these treatments and the diseases which cannot be cured.

This paper is a study based on the above details extracted from the palm-leaf manuscript named *Nayanavithi Vākatam* with No. 8867 of the Manuscript Library in the University of Kerala.

Nayanam means 'eye' and *Vākatam* means 'a book on treatment, in the form of poetry. Since the manuscript explains the 'eye diseases' and their 'treatment methods' in the verse form, it is called *Nayanavithi Vākatam.*

Format of the Manuscript

This manuscript consists of 93 poems with the opening line *Māthumai pākan chonna* (The one who is the half of Umā, the wife of Lord Śiva), sung in the presence of *Mahadoo.*

Evidence

O! Lady with a carp-like eye
With dark thick locks as the nimbus.

It is found that most of the endings of the poems are strong expression such as the quoted poem.

Evidence

Don't do like this/stop to get light.

These are the strong instructions given on the effect of treatment.

Evidence

Sinus will run off without delay (48)
Pain will fly off (39)
Disease will go off clearly (28)

The language format of the manuscript is like this. The following paragraphs give the details of the medical information found in the manuscript.

Nature of a healthy eye

As the manuscript says, a healthy eye should be bright like a moon; the pupil should be like a crystal in the red-lined sclera; the sclera should be pure without any dirt; and the pupil should reflect the image of the viewer. The appearance and size of a healthy eye is also given. The length of the eye ball should be of two inches, breadth of one inch and depth of half an inch.

Causes of Eye-disease

The author narrates the following as causes for eye disease: walking under the hot sun, walking with bare foot under the hot sun, avoiding oil bath, injury, head loading, worrying, excess of intercourse, constipation, depression, walking for a long distance and anger. Besides these, some unavoidable conditions may also cause eye-diseases.

When a man completes 36 years of his life, streaks may appear in the eyes; and they may develop as he grows older. In his old age when he becomes weak then many diseases may affect his eyes in due course.

Classification of Eye-diseases

The author classified the eye-diseases into 96 types. Among the ninety-six diseases, forty-five diseases affect the pupil of the eye, twenty affect the sclera, sixteen the eye-brows and 15 the eye-muscles.

Symptoms of diseases

The symptoms of the affected eyes are: the abnormal dullness of the eye, pain, irritation and pressure. Besides these, the symptoms of some particular diseases are also given in detail.

Parparoham (cataract)

It is the formation of a white layer in the eye which causes struggle in opening the eyes. Little dots may also form in the pupil of the eye which develops dimness and leads even to blindness.

Pillam (Sore eye):

It affects the eyelids and leads to shedding tears, irritation, sensitivity, expelling pus, redness, injured pupil, etc.

The symptoms of diseases like *aruvi neer paichal* (flow of water falls)", "*vellaluthu*" and *Palakuntham* are also revealed separately.

Medicines for Eye-diseases

After diagnosing the nature of disease from its symptoms, medical treatment is given in various forms such as packs, *mathurāthi* balls, dye, tablets and *kulikai* (tablets to be ground with particular fluids). Herbs, roots, gums, metals, non-metals, organs of some animals, minerals and few supplementary medicines are also mentioned in the manuscripts.

Medicinal herbs

More than 50 names of medicinal herbs including licorice, lemon, sesame seeds, cardamom, kacholam, walnut, sandal, dry ginger, *thippili*, basil, *karisulānkanni* are given.

Evidence:

Veppilai thanai araithu veru neyyār kuzhappi kannil
Kāppura vitta pothu kanatthura valiyun theernthu

Seepperu thava murungaiver thāippālil theitthuk
Koppura valaittha pothu kulirnthiru nayananthāne.

The pricking pain in the eye will be relieved when the drops of the mixture of ground neem leaves and ghee are applied in the eye.

Eyes will be cooled and released when a mixture of ground *murungai* root with mother's milk is applied around the eye.

Besides these, roots of lotus and *korai,* gums of *babool* tree, and minerals like 'red soil' are used.

Also, metals and stones like *arappodi,* iron, bronze, copper, copper sulphate, crystal, marble, gold, silver, brass, *kāvikkal* (red stone), *anchanakkal,* and the nine gem stones are used for preparing the medicine.

Along with the above mentioned medicinal items, parts and organs of many living beings such as tortoise shell, the teeth of dog, cow and elephant, elephant tusk, *pumuku chattam* shell, human skull powder, skull of male child, chest bone of chicken and horse's bone are used.

Supplementary medicines like mother's milk, lemon juice, honey, ghee, cow milk, basil juice are also used.

Preparation method

The preparation of medicine by adding proper proportion of medicinal items are explained in detail in the manuscripts.

Evidence

Nālilontākki padham pārtthu,
Eritthurak kāicchi,
Araitthidu nālu chāmam,
Neerilāru chāmam,
Karuppura marunthai yittuk kanatthume poosu mākil
Araitthuap puliyung chukkum athilidu kādi thānum
Eritthurak kāicchik kondu idaiyin meliduvāyāhil
Therippurach chivappu vittuth thelivudan novum pome.

For eye disease and red-eye, boil the ground mixture of tamarind and dry ginger till it becomes black and apply on the eyes. The eye-disease will be cured and eyesight will become clear.

Methods to retain the eyesight

The guidance to be followed in day to day life in order to keep the eyesight clear is given in the manuscripts. It reveals the intimate relation between the eyesight and body hygiene; especially teeth, hands and legs. The methods to maintain hygienic condition of teeth, hands and legs in order to protect our health are also given.

The rinsing methods of cleaning the teeth and thereafter the medicines to be used and the methods of cleaning our limbs and massaging them are also mentioned.

The rinsing methods are *amirtha yoka murai* which stresses on the Sun-worship and then the Moon-worship following a particular method.

Evidence for mouth-rinsing and pure limbs

- Minor eye problems will be cured by cleaning the teeth with hot water. With the cleanliness of teeth, eyesight remains clear even in the old-age.
- Rinsing of the mouth with the mixture of walnut, dry ginger, pepper, *thippili,* rock salt and honey in equal proportion improves the eyesight.
- Washing of the foot by rubbing it on a stone, drying it and then applying pure ghee and sandal paste mixture while drying it under the sun will improve the eyesight.

The method of Amṛtayoga

Wash the hands after meals, take three drops of ghee in hands, rub the hands and apply it in the eyes. Then look at the sun for sometime. It purifies the eyes and works like ambrosia to the eyes.

Conclusion

From the above details, we can understand that the eyesight and health and hygiene of the body are highly related. We have to follow the proverb:

Wash the clothes even if it is rags
Eat after bathing even if it is gruel.

The manuscript *Nayanavithi Vākatam* stresses the importance of protecting our eyes from diseases by cleaning the parts of our body properly and protecting them.

10

Poison Treatment/Anti-Dote Treatment in Tamil Palm-leaf Manuscripts

SENTHIL N.

All living beings on earth love to live a normal healthy life. Man being superior to all living beings identified and discovered ways to diagnose and treat his diseases. The sage Thiruvalluwar says:

One must treat the disease by getting into its very roots, its symptoms, its causes and then prescribe the medicine. (*Thirukkural* 948)

According to this saying, man tends to care his health from birth to death. The result of his concern for his health is the birth of Medical Science. Initially medical treatment was mostly based on natural herbs. In course of time, this form of medical science evolved into many systems such as herbal medicine, Āyurveda, Siddha, Unani, Homoeopathy, and Allopathy.

In order to preserve and keep this life-saving indigenous medical systems, man puts down his findings on palm-leaves. Though a few of them have been destroyed by termites, the remaining palm-leaf manuscripts have proved beneficial to mankind till today. A few of these palm-leaf manuscripts have in them poison-treatment medicines. This paper entitled "Poison treatment/anti-dote treatment in Tamil palm-leaf manuscripts" brings out the details of the diseases caused by poisonous beings, their remedial measures and to suggest methods of treatment as given in the palm-leaf manuscripts.

Poison Treatment Palm-scripts

In the palm-leaf manuscripts that deal basically with different types of poison related diseases, the causes, symptoms and treatment methods have been discussed extensively. They explain the classifications of poison such as plant-poison, poison caused by animal bites, artificial poison, etc. In addition, they give the details of plant-poison caused by eating inedible vegetables and roots and minerals; deadly poison caused by snake-bites and scorpion stings; artificial poison caused by the admixture of chemicals and herbs. The methods to diagnose the type of poison; the treatment methods to be followed; the remedial measures to be taken and the diet to be followed, have been discussed clearly.

The Oriental Research Institute and Manuscripts Library of the University of Kerala have preserved more than thirty of these palm-leaf manuscripts and out of these, *Āruda Nondi*, a poison treatment manuscript is selected here for a detail discussion. This manuscript under the title *Āruda Nondi* with the serial number 6347, is a part of the palm-leaf manuscripts collection in the name *Yoganathar 760 Thirattu.* There is a total of 12 palmleafs in this manuscript which opens with the invocation and concludes with the *Saranam.* The middle portion deals with the names of many poisonous beings, the symptoms of their bites, the treatment to be taken and the medicines to be prescribed.

Poison Treatment

One of the multi-types of poison treatments is *Ahatha Thanthiram* (poison treatment). According to this manuscript, poison is of two types: one is plant-poison and the other is *jaṅgamam,* which are also known as *kṛtrima* poison and *akṛtrima* poison. Of these, plant-poison occurs by eating certain types of tubers and roots. *Jaṅgama* poison occurs due to the poisonous bites of animals like snake, scorpion, spider, centipede and rats.

The symptoms of poison

When a person is affected by the plant-poison or *jaṅgama* poison, symptoms such as body heat, dryness, fainting sensation, weakness, gloom of eyesight, redness in the eyes, irritation, swelling of the body and bleeding occur which lead to a tremendous rise in arthritis and bile secretion that may even be fatal to him.

Poisonous beings

In the poison-treatment manuscript, *Āruda Nondi*, the names of all poisonous animals from snake to lizard have been mentioned with a discussion on the consequent effects of their bites.

Types of snakes

Cobra viper, russells viper, striped racer, carpet viper, rattle snake, sand viper, sand boa, rat snake, etc.

Other small poisonous animals

Goliath spider, scorpion, lady-bird beetle, centipede, chameleon, millipede, dog, mabuya, cougar, monkey, frog, leech, black scorpion, spider, rat, etc.

Reasons for snake bites

Few reasons cited for snake bites are: for food, out of fear, when it is stamped, due to excess of poison, out of anger, out of revenge, on instigation of gods, sages and the God of Death, Yama.

Poison investigation

The presence of poison in a person who is bitten by a snake or an unknown being can be ascertained by the taste of certain bitter-tasting leaves or vegetables. If the body is affected with poison, the bitter leaves and vegetables will taste sweet. If the fingers, nails or hair is pulled, there will not be any pain. The noise in the ears will diminish and eyesight will become dim.

Divisions of cobras

Although snakes are known by many names, they are basically classified into four divisions as Brahma cobra, Kṣatriya cobra, Vaiśya cobra, and Śudra cobra.

Brahma cobra (Brahmin)

This type of snake can be seen in white, red or / and black colours with a shell mark and dots on its hood. Mostly, it inhabits in temples or its surroundings. It raises its hood skywards and dances. It feeds on air, scent of flowers and termaria. On Saturdays and Sundays such snakes can be found roaming outside till 12 o'clock. It usually bites on the right side and aggravates arthritis.

Kṣatriya cobra

This type of snake has colours like dates, grapes and jumplum and its hood has a shell and wheel mark. It normally lives in the hollows of trees. It raises its hood and dances with a balanced view. It feeds on the tuber of *aruham,* insects and rats. It moves around on Saturdays and Mondays during day time. Usually it bites on the left side but rarely on the right which instigates bile secretion.

Vaiśya cobra

The back of this snake has a texture of diamond and topaz with a concoction of red, white and yellow coloured bows like dots. It dwells in houses; and when it raises its hood it dances on all the four directions. It feeds on garden lizards, rats and frogs. During the day-time of Fridays and Tuesdays it can be seen strolling outside. It normally bites on the lefthand side and back of a person.

Śudra cobra

This type of snake has dark wheat complexion and long dots. It inhabits in land-holes and raises its hood and dances facing the earth. It feeds on frogs and fish only on Saturdays and Thursdays. Like the Vaiśya snake, it normally bites on the left and the back.

The disparities in snakes

Although the above mentioned fourfold classification of snakes have different qualities, they can be clubbed together as one, namely the Divine snakes. Under this category, eight different types of snakes are pointed out. They are *Ananthan, Vasuki, Thakan, Kārkodakan, parpan, mahaparpan, chankupālan* and *kulihan.*

The marks of venomous teeth

The teeth of snakes are of four types as: *kāli, kalāśrī, yama* and *yamadūta.* Based on the tooth- marks of one, two, three and four on the bitten part, the snake-bites are known as ¼ bite, ½ bite, ¾ bite and full bite respectively.

The characteristics of snake bite

Venomous tooth	Part of bite	Details of bite	Colour of poison flow	Effect of poison	Treatment method
Kāli	*Pulladi bite*	¼ bite	Like dew	Affect the skin	Chanting *mantra*
Kaalaasthiri	tringle	½ bite	Yellow liquid	Affect the flesh	meditation
Yemen	Like hook	¾ bite	Reddish liquid	Affect the bone	medicine
Yemed-hoothan	Like arrow	Full bite	Blackish liquid	Affect the brain	All the above three

The seat of venom

The whole body of the snake is full of venom like blood is inside a man's body and the secretion of *sukkilam*, the venom inside a snake's body gets activated at the time of the bite and rests under the snake's tooth.

The death point

Snake-bites at certain places in a man's body results in fatal death. The specific places are: head, forehead, eyebrow, chin, lips, chest, palm of hands, breast, armpits, naval, male organs, female organs and the feet.

Stages where snake poison is weak

There are times when deadly poisonous snakes lose the effect of their poison. It usually loses its poison when it is immersed in water, when they are afraid, during fight with mongoose, long move through the woods, due to cold wind, sunshine, when it is sick or hungry or sometimes thirsty and when shedding off skin.

The venom of the Krait cobra

When bitten by a krait cobra, the person becomes completely deaf. Moreover all the above mentioned characteristics of snake bite will simultaneously occur. In order to rid the body of this poisonous toxin, the tuber of *nilappanai* and *uppilankodi* root should be ground well, made into small balls and dried in the shade and administered in the dosage of one ball per day for eight days.

The venom of the Viper snake

There are six types in the viper snake such as gaboon viper, red viper, russels viper, carpet viper, water viper and grass viper. In order to lower the venomous toxin of the viper snake, medicinal treatments such as *nasiam*, smoke, powder, oil and dyes are used.

Medicine

Take the juice of bitter gourd leaf measuring ¼ litre and grind well with pepper and drink on an empty stomach to lower the strength of viper snake bite. In case the poisonous effect is not lowered or the sore snake bite not healed, the bitten person should be given the ground mixture of *veeli* fruit with cow butter to intake.

If there is swelling in the snake bitten part, the roots of *poochimarunthu thakkali* (pest control tomato) and *Nāyuruvi* (devil's horsewhip) should be ground together and applied on the wound.

To control the venom of black viper, the milk of *erukku* (calotropis) and buffalo dung should be ground and applied on the poison affected area.

If a green snake is cut into two pieces and sun-dried and ground with equal proportion of pepper and stored in a bamboo stick and poured into the nose of the bitten man, even the dead body will get up alive.

All the venom of vipers will be controlled when the roots of *kommatti, māthanā, cithuvaraikhodi* and *karanai* are dried and ground together by using a grinding stone and give a quantity of arecanut size to the bitten man.

Common medicine

If you powder the tuber of *pazhupāha*', *chanthi* root, *kāttukkaranai, amukkara, cirukāndhi, soriyetti, marukorai, sānthamām karippāl, oomathuchchāradai, meippeerkkuch cheppu, nerinchi*, *beetle* leaves, *kanavālai, mudakundi* and *veeraikkum* together and add with equal proportion of rice flour and cook and give to the bitten man as food, the poison will lose its effects.

Black scorpion

If this kind of scorpion stings, the stung person will have sweat, bulging of glands, swelling, sensation and his mouth will send out froth. To inactivate this venom, cook *a brinjal* and tie it on the stung part. To remove the venom, a combination of the ground *yettikkāi seed* and *kānchikkāi* should be given by mixing it with honey or droppings of chicken or extract of *beetle* leaves.

Scorpion

To inactivate the venom of scorpion, many methods such as smoke treatment, medicinal bandage, application of medicine and eye- drops can be followed.

Smoke treatment

Smoke the bitten part with the droppings of peafowl or chicken or *seetha chey kazhuneel* root.

Application medicine

Grind beetle leaves and salt and apply on the bitten part; grind the root of *calotropis* and *vānamarunthu* by using the milk of *calotropis* and prepare tablets and apply with hot water on the bitten place. (*Vānamarunthu* is the combination of *vedi*–salt, *sulphur* and *kiri*.)

Bandage medicine

Bandaging the bitten part with crushed leaves of bitter gourd will remove the venom.

Bandaging the bitten part with the ground mixture of *sirukeerai* (a variety of lettuce) and salt will remove the poison.

Spider

These are of white and red colour with stripes at the back. Their venom instigates cough, bile and arthritis. To control this poison, the bitten person should eat the ground root, bark of *sangam* and pepper by mixing it with cow ghee, twice a day.

Beetle Bite

To get rid of the poison of beetle bite, the bitten person

should intake the ground mixture of *veeduch thitthin pattai* and the raw fruit of bay tree eight days.

Dog bite

In order to control the poison of pet dog's bite, there are varieties of treatment methods such as 'application of medicine', 'bandaging treatment' and 'intaking treatment'.

Application treatment

Applying the ground bark of wood-apple tree or applying the ground mixture of tamarind and ant-hill, or the ground mixture of *aeorus*, root of *karunkodi* and garlic with water, can be followed.

Bandaging medicine

Bandaging the bitten part with roasted cotton leaves of light heat; or roasted tamarind leaves; or outer skin of *marukkārai* root with lime; or bandaging with the ground mixture of pepper and the *othiyam* bark are some of the bandaging medicines.

Rat

In the discussion on rat-poison, it is said that there are 18 kinds of rats and their bites will be with different symptoms. Generally, to control the poison of rat-bite, the bitten part should be made sore by applying lime. Then a big size of ground *porusal* bark should be given along with cow ghee for eight days.

The poison will be removed even if the extract of *veliparuthi* is given to drink and is applied on the bitten part.

Giving the *cūraṇa* for a weight of 1¼ *varahan* of asafetida and *seenthil creaper* with beetle leaf extract will inactivate 18 kinds of rat-poison.

Conclusion

Indigenous treatment is the method found out to treat

the disease of man caused by the venom of poisonous beings. The treatments are handled differently based on the day, star, belief, medicine, and nature of their bites. They are used in the form of *cūraṇa* (powder) or tablet or mixture or oil based on the above said factors. Though the medical inventions are in their peak, the ancient method seems to be the apt one even today.

11

Rediscovering the Unique Tradition of Gynaecology and Obstetrics in Kerala based on Manuscripts

P. Vasumathy

"It is not an object to be perceived; nor described, how shall;
I then tell you of it?
You know the mother only if you know the Self" *(Tripura Rahasya)*

"आब्रह्मकीडान्तमिदं निबद्‌घंपुमस्त्रीप्रयोगेन जगत्समस्तम्‌"।
(*Bṛhat Saṁhitā*, 7420.)

(All living things from an ant or worm to Brahma is in one way or other connected and obliged to the female sex)

Introduction

Health care and hence the science of Medicine are of utmost significance to humanity's well-being and survival and takes their inception from Mother Nature. Traditional Indian systems of medicine had been evolved from remote antiquity by people who had a practical insight into the mysteries of nature and harnessed its bounties for the well-being of mankind. Taking its roots from a hoary past, medical wisdom in India was systematized at a slightly later period and has continued to our own period, despite the growing popularity of western medical practice.[1] As we know, the traditional medical systems of India have considered the individual as a whole rather than just a disease. Hence treatment is fine-tuned taking into consideration the individual's constitution, susceptibility to disease, mental makeup, life style and other factors. What is more remarkable about the Indian medical tradition is that it has prevailed at two different levels, namely the classical systems such as Āyurveda, Siddha and Unani and the folk and ethnic systems consisting of several distinct oral and *Nattuvaidya* traditions and tribal practitioners of varied procedure health care and therapy.

The traditional treatment systems of Kerala had developed in an early period even before the advent of the Ayurvedic system from the north. An apt health care system had gradually evolved in this southern region of India through an amalgam of the curing methods of autonomous communities with those imbibed from the intruding Sanskritic Brahmins, Jains, Buddhists, Jews, Christians, and Muslims. The symbiotic process happened mainly between the Sanskritic Ayurvedic traditions of Caraka-Suśruta, the Buddhist Vāghaṭa texts of *Aṣṭāṅgahṛdaya*[2] and *Aṣṭāṅgasaṅgraha* and the *Siddha Cintāmaṇi* traditions with those of the Keralite ethnic traditions and home remedies. Parallel to those, was the utilization of *Sahasrayoga,* a typical Keralite compendium of more than thousand popular formations of household remedies and cures. It would be quite reasonable to think that prior to the propagation of Ayurvedic works in Kerala, there had already existed a more or less developed system of treatment[3] for distressing maladies. Based upon these, along with the Sanskritic and Tamil systems, unique and characteristic treatment modalities were framed in Kerala for Paediatrics, Gynaecology and Obstetrics, Ophthalmology, Toxicology, *Marma* system, *Vṛkṣa Cikitsā* (treatment of trees), *Hastīcikitsā* (treat-ment of elephants) etc. Many of them are specific to the region and indicative of well formulated curative systems that had preceded in Kerala in all these branches of panacea. The authentic tradition of Indian medical thought, especially the South

Indian, the theoretical and practical issues of it, as was formulated several centuries ago, have not yet been presented properly to the modern mind. There are a number of typically Keralite manuscripts and Siddha texts specifically dealing with *Prasūti Tantra* (pregnancy treatments) and *Strīroga* (treatment for afflictions of women).

The present paper is an endeavour to rediscover the unique tradition of Kerala on Gynaecology and Obstetrics and to have a glimpse of its effective contribution to that sphere of medical practice. The study is made based on certain manuscripts on the theme, preserved mainly in the Oriental Institute of Research and Manuscripts Library, University of Kerala. Valuable informations on the subject have also been culled out from a few manuscripts preserved and published by Government Oriental Manuscripts Library, Madras and Government Āyurveda College, Thiruvananthapuram.

Ideas and Practices on Obstetrics and Gynaecology in Indian Traditional Medical texts

Before delving into a description of the manuscripts mentioned above, it would be apt to have a general idea of Obstetrical and Gynaecological knowledge and practices in Indian traditional medical spheres. The study and practice of Obstetrics (*Garbhavijñānam)* depend heavily on the environmental and social factors. It, at the outset, necessitates *Strī Śarīra Vijñānam* or scientific knowledge of the anatomy of woman, physical constitution during different stages of her existence. The term *Strī* is according to *Uṇā Sūtra* derived from the addition of the *pratyaya draṭ* to the root *Stryai* and stands for the place or the living human body where the male sperm (*sukra)* and *strībīja* (*arthava)* can unite and into which the *manojava ātmā* descends to form an embryo and wherein this embryo can further grow and develop into full term foetus. Only the woman's body has been provided with the special organ of *garbhāśaya* (uterus) wherein the union of the sperm and the ovum can take place and lead to the formation of a human being.

In ancient Ayurvedic texts there was no special section on either Obstetrics or Gynaecology though there was one on Paediatrics (*Kumāra-bhṛtya*).[4] This does not however imply that this subject was deliberately omitted. Obstetrics did not generally form a branch of a physician's duty but was handled mainly by midwives or *dāīs* included within the broad, diverse stream of local health traditions, " *the daī(s)* tradition" could be seen as the real mainstream of childbirth care especially for socially, economically and geographically marginalized communities in India.[5] The classical Ayurvedic texts offer a theoretical framework for some of the practices—concepts and languages of *dāīs*, delay in placental delivery and importance of emotional support.[6] Perhaps owing to the social custom of the times, women did not readily seek the help of physicians or surgeons. Both *Caraka* and *Suśruta* discuss the subjects of Obstetrics and Gynaecology at some length in their Saṁhitās, particularly in *śarīra sthāna* and *cikitsā-sthāna.*

Caraka concerns himself mainly with the medical aspects of Gynaecology and with normal pregnancy and delivery. Suśruta deals in addition, with surgical aspects of Obstetrics. If we scrutinize the text of the *Carakasaṁhitā,* available today, its author appears to be a brilliant *prasūti* (delivery) physician. He describes in detail in his *śarīrasthāna* symptoms of a lady in full pregnancy (*Cha. S.* 2.22.4, 16), real labour pain (*Cha. S.* 8.36), the methods and Ayurvedic medicines to reduce the harshness of labour pain (*Ch. S.* 8.38-39), the after delivery care, etc.

Suśruta in *śarīrasthāna* describes how *Jīvātmā* or life principle appears as the twenty fifth principle in the newly formed foetus. The very term *Garbha* denotes the *manojavātma* in the form of *cetanā* (life source) along with the minute atoms of the five elements accepting a new body in the uterus of a woman which is healthy and accepts the union of the *śukra* (sperm) of a healthy father and her own *śoṇita* (ovum). *Suśruta* describes each and every stage of the growth of the foetus in the uterus and the phases of transformation. One most notable aspect is his depiction of the mental relation between the mother and the child in the womb. This type of an affinity which Suśruta depicted two thousand five hundred years ago, has been noted and analysed by Western medicine only very recently. Another famous ancient Indian Ayurvedic compendium the *Kāśyapasaṃhitā* deals principally with the diseases of women and children and their treatment. Miscarriage and related topics on pregnant women are dealt with in a rationalist approach in *Suśruta* and *Caraka,* advising such as bed-rest for women who bleed during early pregnancy and describing how to remove surgically from the womb a baby which has died. By contrast, the Compendium of Kāśyapa approaches the topic of miscarriage from the religious and mythical point of view, presenting a connection with primal legend to explain the genesis of the medical problem.[7]

In *Aṣṭāṅgahṛdaya* and *Aṣṭāṅgasaṅgraha* of Vāgbhaṭa, along with some aspects of *Caraka* and *Suśruta* texts, certain alterations and additions have been made. The traditional Gynaecological texts and practices in Kerala while following Vāgbhaṭa in some fundamentals of Obstetrics and Gynaecology, have provided unique diagnosis and medicinal preparations of their own. This fact is clear not only in the Keralite treatises of *Sahasrayoga* and *Cikitsāmañjarī,* but also in the numerous treatises composed by the traditional *vaidyas* (physicians) of Kerala.

Contributions of Kerala

The history of the local medical traditions of Kerala can be deduced from *Maṇipravāla* literature (a mixture of Malayalam and Sanskrit) of the fourteenth, fifteenth and sixteenth centuries. The great *Ācāryas* of Āyurveda in Kerala applied very effective *yogas* (special preparative modes of medicines) from generation to generation. The *yogas* of the indigenous medicine are described in works like *Sahasrayoga* (thousand medicinal preparations). It is a great contribution of Kerala to the world of Āyurveda and is a codification of many of the traditional medicines of Kerala. It includes descriptions of problems and maladies related to Obstetrics and Gynaecology. The text is followed not only by traditional physicians but by people and families all over Kerala. The medicinal *yogas* prescribed in the *Sahasrayoga* like *Kasturyādī*, *Gorocanādī*, *Kombañjādī* and *Dhanvaṇtaram* are alien to Sanskrit Ayurvedic texts. The last one is especially practised during pregnancy and after delivery.

Cikitsāmañjarī is another typical Kerala treatise on medicinal practices. It is an original work by Pulamantol Muss, one of the *Aṣṭavaidyas*. There are unique and special preparations of medicines for Obstetrical and gynaecological purposes like the one given to a woman for fever after-delivery women.

Bṛhaccharīram of P.S Varier contains an elaborate appendix to *Garbhavakrantiyam* and *Sarira* of *Aṣṭāṅgahṛdaya*. Here an attempt is made to co-ordinate Āyurveda with modern science. Similarly *Vaidyamanoramā* in Sanskrit, is a text of purely Kerala origin and very popular among the physicians of Kerala. Two other important medical works of Kerala related to Obstetrics and Gynecology are *Garbharakṣākrama* and *Vaidya Vijñāna* authorized by Mahākavi Vallathol.

Manuscripts on Obstetrics and Gynaecology

While we delve into the contents of many of the original manuscripts mentioned above on the themes of Obstetrics and Gynaecology in Kerala, it can be concluded that these typical Kerala pıeparations had been used through ages by the traditional Vaidyas of the region for treatments related to *Strīroga* (treatment for maladies affecting women), *Prasūti Tantra* (pregnancy treatment) and *Sūtikāroga* (diseases affecting women post-delivery). For example, one of the most popular and typically Malayalee manuscripts appears to be that entitled *Garbhacikitsā*. Four versions of the treatise are kept in the ORI and Manuscripts Library, University of Kerala.[8] This old Malayalam manuscript deals with treatment relating to Obstetrics and Gynecology which the ancient physicians of Kerala found efficacious by experience. Though the title *Garbhacikitsā* is given to this work, its content includes details of menstrual periods, conception, pre-natal care, treatment after childbirth, detailed descriptions of the symptoms, causes and treatment of certain infantile diseases (especially *Karappaṇ*).

Similar in content as the aforesaid manuscript is an old Malayalam work with the same title *Garbhacikitsā* found and published from Government of Oriental Manuscripts Library, Madras in 1949.[9] The title *Garbhacikitsā* is given to this work probably because it deals with the treatment from the time of conception upto the growth of the child. The personal details of the author of the work remains enveloped in obscurity. The descriptions of various diseases and remedies are almost invariably found in what are called *matiris* popular among the inidigenous *Vaidyas.* One can therefore, only say that this must have been one of the old books kept in strict secrecy by traditional family practitioners. What strikes us is the similarity in diagnosis of diseases pertaining to conceiving of women, infants' treatment details and special *yogas* between this manuscript and the four similarly titled manuscripts preserved in ORI and Manuscripts Library of Kerala University.

Despite the fact that the ailments and remedies dealt with are written in consonance with the system of Āyurveda, many of the diseases and *Mūlikas* (herbs) spoken of here are not to be seen even in the famous Ayurvedic works as those of Caraka, Suśruta and Vāgbhaṭa. For instance, symptoms of many infantile diseases like different varieties of *Karappaṇ* and their treatments depicted in this text do not find a place in well known Ayurvedic works. So also some medicines and herbs such as *Mūtayinha, Kallatinayakam, Kakkakodi,*

Kizhukkila, Koppiliyila etc are not found in those texts. The description of diseases and their treatment as well as the Tamil mixed Malayalam language used in the manuscript would in fact lead one to the conjucture that these might have been taken from *Siddhavaidya* or *Cintāmaṇi Vaidya.* In this connection a pertinent question might well be asked. How then can the description of diseases like *Karappaṇ* etc. be seen in books like *Ārogyakalpadruma, Ārogyacintāmoṇi* etc printed in the early years in Malabar? The explanation offered is that information taken from old manuscripts like *Garbhacikitsā* would have been converted into Sanskrit and Malayalam verses and printed with modification.[10]

There are six sections in this very useful and practical manuscript. The first part gives details on menses, conception, abortion, diseases affecting pregnant women etc., the second chapter is titled *Bālanidānam* and deals with conditions of newly born babies and is a general pediatrics manual and the third part contains medicinal preparations for infantile diseases and methods of their application. The fourth section of the treatise is a detailed description of the growth and problems of children from the first month of their birth to the twelfth and then yearly occurring maladies and their solutions upto the sixteenth year. The fifth chapter is an indepth diagnostic presentation of infantile disease, varieties of *Karappaṇ.* Detailed symptomatic cures of varied diseases affecting women and especially expecting and post-natal women form the subject matter of the sixth and the last section of the manuscript *Garbhacikitsā.*

On an ultimate analysis it would become clear that the maladies and their cures explained in this text are not based upon the *Tridoṣa Siddhānta* of Āyurveda. Nevertheless it may be asserted that it follows certain traditional aspects of child disease and their cure. Many of the herbs are peculiar to this part of the country and the efficacy of most of the medicinal preparations appears to be time tested by the Vaidya authors on personal experience. From the language used in the text it may be concluded that the traditional ethnic Vaidyas of Kerala having some knowledge of Āyurveda and Tamil Siddha systems might have evolved their own diagnostic and treatment modes for problems in Obstetrics and Gynaecology.

Other Manuscripts

Of the other manuscripts on the subject preserved in ORI and Manuscripts Library, Kerala, three copies of the text titled *Garbharakṣavidhikal*[11] written in Malayalam are conspicuous manuals on *Sūtikā Vijñānam*. They contain systematic regimen to be followed during pregnancy, delivery and post-natal conditions. Besides common Ayurvedic knowledge, many typical Keralite *yogas*, practices, medications, oil preparations and their use during pregnancy and delivery and in *Sūtikā-avasthā* (post-natal condition) of women are provided in *Garbharakṣāvidhikal* (systematic protection and preservation of the foetus and the *Sūtikā*).

Another significant manuscript from the same source related to the subject is titled *Garbhalakṣaṇam.*[12] The manuscript is primarily an astrological text with indications to assess the symptoms of pregnancy, determination of the sex of the child, indications of imminent delivery etc. Though some religious and astrological beliefs are mixed with scientific diagnosis, it is a typical text of an indigenous system of prognostication on valuable medical aspects.

There are two manuscript volumes of the text titled *Prasavacikitsā*[13] in Malayalam in ORI and Manuscripts Library, University of Kerala. It contains many preparations of oil, *Kaṣāya* (a systematically prepared decoction of herbs and roots), *ghṛta* (medicinal ghee, prepared as per specific dictum) etc to be administered to the pregnant woman before and after delivery. Many of these are typically Keralite, made out of ingredients unique to the region and most effective for easy delivery and efficient post-natal care.

A much more notable treastise on the subject of Obstetrics

and Gynaecology kept in the same repository, is the one titled *Garbhāvakrāntiyum Cikitsavidhikālam* rendered in Malayalam.[14] In Ayurvedic classics the *ātmā* (soul) in accordance with the *karma* (actions) of its *pūrva janma* (past life) enters the uterus, joins or gets united with the ovum and sperm and together make the *jivātmā* in the form of *garbha* (the fertilized ovum coming down the fallopian tube) and reach the uterus. The method of attaining this *garbhāvasthā* or condition of being born as a foetus by the *Cetana adhiṣṭita mahābhūta* (life producing great element) is referred to as *garbhāvakrānti.* The *Garbha avakrānti* is the reproduction of life which of course is remarkable. In this process the two nuclei (male and female) fuse together and the normal DNA is synthesized. These whole process or changes may be the entry or *avakramaṇam* of *manojava ātmā,* said in classics.[15]

The aforesaid text contains the details about the process of *garbha avakrānti* and the regimen for *garbhinī Vyavasthā* (antenatal care). Very effective treatment modes for a number of diseases in connection with pregnancy, delivery and post-natal care are systematically provided. Typical and unique medications and *yogas* of Kerala form part of the panacea presented in the manuscript like *Nārikelarasayanam, Narikelathaila* to be used as *sneha dravya* according to *Satmya, Kalyanagulam, Drāshadi, Kurunthotikashayam* etc. In short, it is a very precious treatise on Obstetrics and Gynaecology, written in verses in Malayalam language.

Effective panacea for infertility due to various reasons was known to Kerala physicians. One of the valuable treatises kept in ORI and ML of Kerala University titled *Vandhyatāchikitsa*[16] in Malayalam deals with the causes of infertility and possible treatments. The causative factors for infertility are keenly analysed in the treatise and treatments with specially Keralite medications, medicinal *yogas* and single herb cures like *tiruthali* etc. are prescribed for curing the problems related to infertility.

Besides the above mentioned treatises, a number of manuscript texts on Paediatrics, *Jyotiṣa* (Astrology) and Tantra preserved in the same venerable repository also have sections on Obstetrics and Gynaecology. Unique formation of remedies and single herbal cures known and traditionally practised by Kerala Vaidyas for generations are revealed through these manuscripts on various subjects.

Manuscripts published by the Patent Cell of the Directorate of Āyurveda Medical Education

The patent cell functioning in the Directorate of Āyurveda Medical Education, Government of Kerala since the year 2003 has published some deciphered manuscripts for the benefit of Āyurveda fraternity. The Cell has already collected more than thousand manuscripts and has started digitizing them with the help of Central Government Ayush Department. The first volume titled *Keralīya Oushadha Vijñānam* has brought out four of the manuscripts.[17] The palm leaf manuscripts contain several medicinal preparations intended for *Strīrogacikitsā, garbha-cikitsā,* treatment for fibroids, *Sūtikācikitsā, bālacikitsā* (paediatric treatments) etc. The innumeral prescriptions for preparation of *auṣadha yogas,* stipulations for diagnosis of diseases and the methods of medicinal applications etc are given in simple verses in a Sanskrit and Tamil mixed Malayalam. There are many prescriptions for preparation and application of *Siddha* medicines in the form of different types of *bhasmas.*

Brief analysis of native medical texts on Obstetrics and Gynaecology

Besides the above mentioned manuscripts and palm leaf treatises on Obstetrics and Gynaecology umpteen numbers of them are kept obscure due to ignorance or guarded off under private custody. Much of the native knowledge in this as well as in other aspects of Ayurvedic and Siddha system of cure have come out through the practitioners and through various *Vaidyā* texts authored by eminent physicians several years. Many of them are compendiums of conclusive cures for all types of maladies, whereas some of them deal specifically with Obstetrics, Gynaecology and Paediatrics. One of the earliest of such texts is the treatise titled *Cūtaka Nūl* in Tamil authored by Siddha Saint Yoohimuni. It tells us about nineteen kinds of diseases of the uterus and methods to avoid infertility. Just like Toxicology and Ophthalmology, Gynaecology and Paediatrics received great attention through Kerala physicians and a major contributions were made. Certain communities like the Veleppanikkan, the Kaniyan, the Warrier, the Ezhavas etc produced expert practitioners in Gynaecology and Paediatrics. Besides many members of elite castes like the Warrier, the Kṣatriyas, the Nairs, etc. have contributed specialized treastises on different branches of medical practices like *Kalpadrumam* of Kaikulangara Rama Warrier, *Karappaṉ* by Kunjikuttan Thampuran, *ārogyacintāmaṇī, Garbhārakṣākrama* and *Vaidyajīvana* by Vallathol Narayana Menon belong to this category. The *yogas* (special preparative medicine) specific to Kerala, described in works like *Sahasrayoga* (thousand yogas) include some unique medical fusion like *Dhanvantaram, Gorocanādi, Kasturyādi, Kombañjādi,* etc. which are alien to Sanskrit Ayurvedic texts. Of these medicated oils like *Dhanvanthara, Kṣīrabālā taila* etc. are special medicines for women in pregnancy and after delivery.

Malayalam texts deal in general with ailments, their symptoms, causes, cures, medicinal preparations and their application regimen, while many of them contained Obstetric and gynaecological aspects as well. In this series come texts like *Cikitsamañjarī, Cikitsāsaṁgraha, Cikitsāsāram, Nidanavum cikitsayum* preserved in ORI and ML at Thiruvananthapuram. *Cikitsāmañjarī* is an orginal work by Pulamantol Moss, one of the famous *Aṣṭavaidyas* and the author of *Kairali. Kairali* is popularly known as Putamantol commentary on *Aṣṭāṅgahṛdaya* and is an authoritative work on many aspects of Ayurvedic practices. Indu who wrote *Śaśilekha,* the commentary on *Aṣṭāṅgahṛdaya* and *Aṣṭāṅgsaṅgraha* belonged to Kerala. *Vaidya manoramā* is in Sanskrit and purely of Kerala origin. It is very popular among the physicians of Kerala.

Sūtikāmṛtam is a Vaidya text in verse written in Malayalam and composed by one of the great Ayurvedic scholars of Kerala, Kayikkara P.M. Govindan Vaidyan.[18] It was published during the year 1910 and contained twelve chapters dealing with aspects like the correct routine, *doṣādivijñānam, putrakamīyam, garbholpatī, garbharakṣā, prasavācāra* (the regimen during delivery), *garbhāvyapat* (problems during pregnancy), *prasavavaiṣamyam* (troubles of delivery), *bālaparicāraṇam* (care of the new born), *bālarogacikitsā* (treatment of diseases affecting children), *auṣadhakalpanam* etc. In short it is a popular treatise and subjects of interest to all mothers and would be mothers like *Sūtikarma, Garbharakṣā,* paediatrics etc. There are a number of other known and unknown texts and practices, native to Kerala and which provide valuable addition to knowledge on Obstetrics and Gynaecology. In more recent times the *Bṛhaccharīram* of Vaidyaratna P.S. Warrier, the famous Ayurvedic physician and entrepreneur in Kerala, provides an elaborate appendix to *garbhāvakrāntiyam* and *Śarīra* of *Aṣṭāṅgahṛdaya* and co-ordinates Āyurveda with modern science.[19]

In short, the subject of *prājāpatyam* i.e. the promotion of life through the creation of children and keeping up of the divinity of family life, was seen as the prime duty by the Keralites. Keeping in tune with this idea from the time of the Vedic saṁhitās to *Bṛhaccharīram,* details of time tested knowledge on *garbhādhāna* (conception), the relation between, prakṛti, puruṣa, the five elements, the soul, mind, God and the *jīvātmā's* entry into the mother's womb during particular junctures of *garbhasambhava,* the dictums for the attainment of the best child, evolution and care of the embryo and the expectant mother, month by month symptoms of imminent delivery, preparation of *Sūtikagṛha* (delivery home) methods of easy delivery, the diseases affecting the pregnant and delivering woman, *Kaumārabrātya* (child care and mother's protection), *Kṣīradoṣasaṁśodhana* (methods of abundant production and the avoiding of diseases affecting breast milk), cures for maladies affecting the newly born children as well as the feeding mothers, paediatrics in short) and *Sūtikāroga* and care in general had been discussed in the vaidya manuscripts and texts of Kerala as in the classical works of India like *Carakasaṁhitā, Suśruta Saṁhitā, Kāśyapa saṁhitā,* etc.

There had been physicians and ethnic curers in Kerala interested in recording and publishing their clinical experience, regardless of the results of the treatment. They had been doing it in the best interest of the transference of their practical knowledge to the succeeding generations. Many of these treatises contain down to earth practical guidelines to the practitioners and ample materials for research scholars.

Specimens of typical Kerala prescriptions on Obstetrics and Gynaecology

As mentioned earlier, there are a number of unique and typical guidelines for regimen and *yogas* for women in Kerala, the knowledge of which was transferred through generations. Local prescriptions for pregnant women, like the smearing of oil, taking of medicated ghee and tamarind juice etc at proper periods of pregnancy endorse health and happiness not only for the mother, but to the baby as well.[20] Some such distinct oils, ghee, *lehya* etc. mentioned in the manuscripts and Vaidya texts of Kerala or continued to be prepared and applied through generations as home remedies are *Kṣīrabālā taila* (oil), *Candanādi taila, Piṇḍataila,* etc. are special formulations of oil for heat rushes during menopause or after hysterectomy. *Kurundūṭikaṣāya* (decoction of *saida retussa* with milk) is taken by pregnant women from the fifth month for easy delivery. *Dhanvantaram* oil is to be applied by expecting mothers for swiftness of the body and relieving of joints pain etc. *Thengumpūkkulalehyam* prepared out of the flower bunch of the coconut tree with appropriate herbs, has to be taken in prescribed measure for menstrual problems, for the retrieval of the general health of women after delivery, for dispelling backache and also for enhancing the quantity of breast milk in feeding mothers. A slightly different preparation modality is applied in the making of *Thenginpūkkula Rasāyana* which is also used as a therapeutic remedy for women in confinement; *Vasundharākaplam,* an effective cure for many diseases connected with heat and unhealthy discharges in women; *Kuriñjikuzhampu,* a *lehya* medical formulation made with the medicinal herb, *Kuriñji (barleria priyanittis lin)* as the main ingredient, administered to women immediately after delivery to rejuvenate their health and to cure the injuries; *Cuvannullikehyam* (a preparation out of small onion and some slight herbs) administered for the restoration of health of women after delivery and also *Ajamāṁsarasāyana* (special medicated formulation with mutton juice as the main ingredient) used for the same purpose. Besides these immunerable ethnic treatments, herbs and grandma's cures are adhered to through generations of Keralites in the preservation of the health of women and children and especially before, during and after delivery. In this context it can be called for how the *daśapuṣpa* (the ten herbs and flowers) used by Malayalee women as part of their *Thiruvathira festival,* many of them have curative traits in women-related maladies.

Uterine fibroid is a fairly common gynae problem which causes a lot of discomfort to the sufferer. Ayurvedic douche with herbal decoctions helps to reduce the size of the utrine fibroid considerably. It is likely to be more effective if done in the initial stages. Ayurvedic manuscripts speak of the general judicial administering of medicines which are routinely administered for the treatment of *Antra-vidradhi* like uterine fibroid. Physicians in Kerala have advocated along with oral medications, douche with *Aśvathapatra/tvak* (leaves and barks of *ficus religiosa*) and *kvātha,* to be done on a regular basis. Such Ayurvedic methods, it is argued can gradually reduce and even do away with uterus fibroid and thus surgical intervention can be avoided.[21]

Besides such manuscripts, Vaidya texts and articles, ethnic prescriptions etc. some of the great socio-religious reformers of modern Kerala like Śrī Nārāyaṇa Guru and Cattambi Svamikal have contributed greatly to the development of traditional treatment systems. Narayana Guru has especially made valuable contribution related to Obstetrics and Gynaecology through his dictums published in the text *Śrī Nārāyaṇadharmam.*[22]

Conclusion

A perusal of the precious Ayurvedic and Siddha manuscripts in Kerala on the domain of Obstetrics and Gynaecology provides valuable insights into the very creation and existence of human kind through the medium of woman as mother. Further as surmised earlier, even before the advent of Sanskrit or Pali Ayurvedic traditions from the North, Kerala had her own unique and effective treatment modalities based on written and unwritten texts and oral knowledge passed on to them by ancestors. It can no doubt be surmised that the local systems and practices in Gynaecology and Obstetrics, as in certain other departments of health preservation, cure of maladies and therapeutics must have influenced the structure and content of Āyurveda in general and in turn helped its further progress in Kerala.

References

1. Vidyalankara. S.K. Ramachandra Rao (ed.), *Encyclopaedia of Indian Medicine,* vol. 2, Popular Prakashan, Mumbai, rept. 2005.

2. There are differences of opinion about the idea whether Vāgbhaṭa, the Indian physician of AD fourth century was the author of both *Aṣṭāṅgahṛdya* and *Aṣṭāṅgasaṅgraha.* From various internal and external evidences it has been surmised so. Vide Lilly Sankunni, *Auruedam* (Mal.), State Institute of Language, Kerala, Trivandrum, 1988. One strong view is that Vāgbhaṭa I (*Vriddha* Vāgbhaṭa), was the composer of *Aṣṭāṅgasaṅgraha* and Vāgbhaṭa II who compiled *Aṣṭāṅgahṛdaya* has clearly stated in *Uttarasthāna* that his, treatise is based on the compilation of *Vṛddha* Vāgbhaṭa; G. Kuppuram, "A Survey of the history of Medicine in Ancient India," V.K. Thakur and K.K. Mandal (ed.), *Science Technology and Medicine in Indian History,* p. 96, Janaki Prakasan, New Delhi, 2000.
3. C.N. Krishnankutty Varier, *History of Āyurveda,* Aryavaidyasala, Kottakkal, 2005.
4. P. Kutumbiah, *Ancient Indian Medicine,* Orient Longman, Hyderabad, rept. 1999, p.177.
5. Mira Sadgopal, "Can Maternity Services open upto the Indigenous Traditions of Midwifery?", *Economic and Political Weekly,* vol. XLIV, no.16, April 2000, p. 54.
6. Ibid., cited from Chawla, Janet, "Child bearing and culture: Dai as Ritual Practitioner", *Journal of Indian Social Institute,* New Delhi, 1994; A Singh, "Her one foot in this world and one in the other: Āyurveda, Dais and Maternity", Chawla, ed., *Birth and Birth Givers,* New Delhi, 2006.
7. Dominick Wujastyk, *The Roots of Āyurveda, Selections from Sanskrit Medical Writings,* Penguin Books, New Delhi, 2001, pp. 208-9.
8. Oriental Research Institute and Manuscripts Library, University of Kerala is a repository of more than sixty-five thousand palmleaf manuscripts of which above two thousand are medical treatises including texts on Obstetrics and Gynecology; of the manuscripts titled *garbhacikitsā,* the four of them series no. 2455, *grantha* no.1200, reg. no. T. 1544; also see series no. 2452, *grantha* no. 120, reg. no. 16548; series no. 2454, *grantha* no.1000, reg. no. 18746 preserved in ORI nd ML, Trivandrum. The MSS were collected from different persons like K.V. Manalikkara, Mantravadi Krishnanpotti, the family repositories of Thekkepushpakam, Marathumpilli, etc.
9. The manuscript from Oriental Manuscripts Library, Madras, entitled *Garbhachikitsa* is critically edited with introduction and notes by Dr. N. Madhava Menon, Madras Government Oriental Series, no. XX, Madras, 1949.
10. Ibid., N. Madhava Menon, the editor of the published Manuscript has opined so, after detailed and comparative study. Madhav Menon was Professor of Āyurveda, College of Indian Medicine, Madras.
11. *Garbharakṣāvidhikāl* (Mal.), MSS, series no. 2456, reg. no. 16655, series

no. 2457, reg. no. 16656, series no. 2458, reg. no. 20072, series no. 2459, reg. no. 1194 –A, ORI and ML, KU, Trivandrum, collected from Kilimanoor palace, Kilimanoor and H.H. The Maharaja's Palace Library, Trivandrum.

12. *Garbhalakṣaṇam* (Mal.), MSS, reg. nos. C565 and 1495, ORI and ML, KU, Trivandrum, collected from Paliam Estate, Kochi.
13. *Prasavacikitsā* (Mal.), MSS, series no. 5135, reg. no. 4120, series no. 5136, reg. no.17103, ORI and ML, KU, Trivandrum.
14. *Garbhavakrantiyam Cikitsavidhikālam* (Mal.), MSS, ser.no.2462, Grantha no. 770, reg. no. 1142, ORI and ML, KU, Trivandrum; collected from the family of Edayavanathu.
15. *"Sukraśoṇitam garbhāṣayasthānam ātmaprikriti vikara sammoorchitam ethyuchyate", Śuśruta Saṁhitā* 5/3, *Aṣṭāṅga Saṁgraha,* 2/1 Indu.
16. *Vandhyatā Cikitsā* (Mal.), MSS, series no.7238, reg. no.1464, ORI and ML, KU, Trivandrum.
17. *Keralīya Ouṣadha Vijñānam* (Mal.), vol. 1, Patent Cell, Directorate of Āyurveda Medical Education, Government of Kerala, Thiruvananthapuram, 2009. The ensuing volumes based on manuscripts are under the process of being published.
18. Lilly Sankunny, *Āyurveda Ithihāsam* (Mal.), p. 115. Kayikkara Govindan Vaidyan was a great Sanskrit scholar and had attained the title of *Abhinavavagbhata* from the renowned Malayalam poet Kumaranasan.
19. N.V. Krishnankutty Varier, *History of Āyurveda,* Arya Vaidya Sala, Kottakkal, 2005.
20. K.K.N. Kurup and K. Vijayakumar, "The Evolution of Indigenous Health Tradition of Kerala", *Science, Technology and Medicine in Indian History,* p. 386, Janaki Prakashan, New Delhi, 2000.
21. Dr. P.K. Warier, "Note on Clinical Experience", *Global Āyurveda,* vol.1, no. 6, Global Media India, Kochi, August-September, 2005.
22. Swami Sreenarayana Theerthar (ed.), *Śrīnārāyaṇadharmam* (Mal.), SNDS Trust, Publication Division, Sivagiri, 2005.

12

Systems of Medicine in Tantra Manuals of Kerala

S.A.S. Sarma

Kerala has had, from early times, a continuous and comparatively rich tradition of scientific and technical advances, as evidenced by the volume of literature on these disciplines presently available to us, mostly in the form of palm leaf manuscripts. The major scientific disciplines, which have been depicted in the literature produced in Kerala, are Tantra, Āyurveda and Jyotiṣa.

Most of the Tantric texts produced in Kerala confine themselves to the *Kriyā* and *Caryā*, relating to temple worship and religious rites; and they are multi-oriented as different deities are worshipped in the land, in contrast to limiting themselves to one school and one deity. But, there are certain other texts of Kerala, which deal not only with rituals but with topics other than rituals, such as architecture, iconography, toxicology, treatment for insane, treatment for different kinds of fevers, treatment for children's diseases, infertility, etc.

The *Īśānagurudevapaddhati* of Īśānagurudeva, *Yogaratnāvalī* of Śrīkaṇṭha, *Tantrasārasaṅgraha* of Nārāyaṇa and *Prayogasāra* of Govinda could be taken as examples of the above mentioned type. This paper will discuss some of the topics related to the systems of medicine discussed in the above mentioned four manuals.

Systems of Medicine dealt with in the early Tantra Manuals

As attested by the early Śaiva texts the basic Tantra texts came out of the Īśāna face of Sadāśiva and the Tantras such as *Bhūtatantras* and *Garuḍatantras*, came out of the other four faces of Sadāśiva, namely, Sadyojāta, Vāmadeva, Aghora and Tatpuruṣa. While the Bhūtatantras are exclusively concerned with curing poisons and related illnesses, the *Gāruḍika* texts are concerned with the classifications of snakes, treatment of snakebite, and illnesses caused by other venomous creatures. The unpublished *Kriyākālaguṇottara* is an early Śaiva text that combines these two groups. In the beginning of this text, Kārtikeya asks Īśvara to explain him in detail the following topics:

vividhaṃ me śrutaṃ tantraṃ loke āścaryakārakam /
siddhimuktipradaṃ sarvaṃ tvayoktaṃ parameśvara //
na śrutaṃ gāruḍaṃ kiñcit sadyaḥ pratyayakārakam /
tamācakṣva suraśreṣṭha mama bhaktasya śaṅkara //
lakṣaṇaṃ nāgajātīnāṃ garbhotpattimaśeṣataḥ /
rūpakaṃ sarvanāgānāṃ vyantarāṇāṃ ca jātakam //
grahayakṣapiśācānāṃ śākinīṇāṃ ca lakṣaṇam /
bālagrahāśca ye krūrāḥ pīḍyante nityanirghṛṇāḥ //
nārīgarbhakarā ye tu teṣāṃ kathaya rūpakam /
gonasānāṃ tu deveśa vṛścikānāṃ tu lakṣaṇam //
anye 'pi vividhā duṣṭā rāsabhāḥ kīṭalūṭayaḥ /
jvarāśca katidhā proktā asādhyasādhyameva ca //
jñānayogakriyādīkṣāmantrāścācāryalakṣaṇam /
dīkṣitāṇaṃ ca samayāsiddhisādhanasādhake //
gāruḍaṃ bhaktatantraṃ ca siddhāntaṃ yacca uttamam /
ekatra saṃsthitaṃ sarvaṃ kathayasva prasādataḥ //[1]

Khaḍgarāvaṇa, Kālakūṭa, Trottala, Trottalottara, Devatrāsa, Sugrīva are some of other early texts of Tantra which belong to the group of *Bhūta/Gārūḍatantras.*

The four Kerala ritual manuals which we mentioned earlier follows the scheme of *Kriyākālaguṇottara* by dealing with topics that are discussed generally in the manuals of Bhūtatantra and Gāruḍatantra.

It is worth to note here that Vāsudeva, a Kerala commentator in his commentary on the *Tantrasārasaṅgraha* quotes the *Kriyākālaguṇottara*, which shows that the Kerala authors of Tantra literature might have been aware of this early text.

The Kearla ritual texts that deals with the systems of Medicine—A brief Introduction

(1) Īśānaśivagurudevapaddhati: The text consists of nearly18000 stanzas in various metres and is divided into a total of 119 palmleaves of varying length. It is divided into four parts, namely (i) *Sāmānyapāda* (ii) *Mantrapāda* (iii) *Kriyāpāda* and (iv) *Yogapāda.* Apart from dealing with rituals the text deals with the application for averting the evil effects of poison; malicious plants and diseases; the use of medicines; the properties of medicinal herbs; the science of magic, etc.[2] We could see that in the following verses the text introduces the topics related to treatments:

viṣagrahāmayārtīnām iti pūrvaṃ pradarśitam /
vastunirdeśapaṭale yasmāt tattataḥ kathyate //
abhivandya guruṃ tatra nāgāṅścānantapūrvakam /
saṃkṣipya viṣatantrebhyo lokānāṃ hitakāmayā//
vol. II, 39.1-2

atha grahacikitsātra likhyate nātivistṛtā /
tatra bālacikitsāyāḥ prakārā bahudhā smṛtāḥ //
teṣvādau matamāśritya khaḍgarāvaṇacoditam /
*nārāyaṇīyoditaṃ ca mārgadvayam ihocyate//*vol. II, 41:1-2

(2) *Tantrasārasaṅgraha: The Tantrasārasaṅgraha of Nārāyaṇa* is a digest on the cure of poison and worship of certain deities and some of the worship included there are meant for magical purposes. Taking into consideration of the first ten chapters dealing with *viṣa* and the author being

Nārāyaṇa it is also called as *Viṣanārāyaṇīya*. The author appears to give the title *Tantrasārasaṅgraha* for his work, as is evident from the line '*Śikhāyogāditantrebhyaḥ kriyate sārasaṅgrahaḥ*'. From this reference it is clear that the author has used the *Śikhā* and *yoga* Tantras as source for this text:

yāvatsāmarthyam asmābhiḥ sarvalokahitaiṣibhiḥ /
śikhāyogāditantrebhyaḥ kriyate sārasaṅgrahaḥ // 1:2 //

The *Tantrasārasaṅgraha* containing thirty-two chapters and about 2100 verses besides the mantra portions is a text on *Viṣavaidya, Mantravāda* and *Tantra.* The first ten chapters of the text are devoted to the *viṣavaidya* or toxicology. Next four chapters give an account of the subject *grahapīḍās* including the mental disease (*unmāda)* and their treatment. Chapters fifteen and sixteen provide the bodily ailments and *Tāntrika* treatment for them. Chapters seventeen and eighteen give a description of *kṣudraprayoga* and its remedies. Chapter nineteen is devoted to the Vinodaprayoga-s. Chapters twenty to thirty-two deals on the *Kāmika-karmas*.

The *Tantrasārasaṅgraha* includes the following topics namely, *viṣacikitsā, grahadoṣaparihāra, rogopakrama, kṣudropādhiśamana, narmakarmāṇi* and *kāmyaprayoga* which come under the *ṣaṭkarma* as defined by the text:

viṣagrahāmayadhvaṃsāḥ kṣudraṃ narma ca kāmikam /
iti ṣaṭkārmikaṃ tantram etat siddhidvayāspadam // 1:3 //

The author himself claims that his text contains all the topics related to *ṣaṭkarma* and feels happy of compiling such a text thus:

ṣaṭkarmāṇyakhilāni naiva kathitānyekatra tatsaṃgrahāt /
tuṣṭiḥ syād viduṣām iti sphuṭadhiyā tantraṃ mayaitat kṛtam//
32:68 //

The *Tantrasārasaṅgraha* follows the *Īśānagurudevapaddhati* while discussing certain topics.[3]

(3) *Yogaratānvali:* The unpublished *Yogaratānvali* of Śrīkaṇṭhaśambhu contains nine chapters and deals with different kinds of poisonous stings, snakes and snake bites, treatment for different type of fever, rituals related to *Tripurā,* Alchemy, methods for preparing fruit syrups, etc. The text refers to twelve famous works on *Viṣatantra*:

pakṣirājaṃ śikhāyogaṃ bindusāraṃ śikhāmṛtam /
tottalaṃ kālakūṭaṃ ca kṛṣṇāgaṃ tottalottaram //
kaṭāhaṃ chāgatuṇḍaṃ ca sugrīvaṃ karkaṭāmukham /
etāni viṣatantrāṇi dvādaśāvocadīśvaraḥ // 1:4-5 //

(4) *Prayogasāra:* Another unpublished ritual manual, the *Prayogasāra* of Govinda written in the same style as *Tantrasārasaṅgraha* by one Govinda contains two parts namely *tantrabhāga* and *auṣadhabhāga.* While the first part deals with rituals related to different deities, the second part deals with topics such as poison treatment, cure for different types of disease, *yoga,* treatments for infertility, methods for protecting the foetus, methods for protecting a child from *bālagraha,* treatment for insane, treatment for different types of poison, treatment for different types of fever etc.

ādau praṇamya sarvajñān gurūnājñāprabodhakān/
prayogasāraṃ vakṣyāmi nānāvijñānasādhanam//
tantrasāraṃ samālocya svasāmarthyānurūpataḥ/
bālānāṃ bodhasidhyartham kriyate sārasaṅgrahaḥ// 1:2 //

Some of the important topics on systems of medicine discussed in the Kerala ritual manuals

Toxicology: The traditional method of treatment for poisoning in Kerala is classified broadly into two categories, namely *Viṣavaidya* and *Viṣavidyā.* The former, *Viṣavaidya* is pure medical practice using medicinal plants and mineral drugs while the latter, *Viṣavidyā* includes recitation of mantras and ritual practices in the process of treatment for poisoning. Even though Caraka and Suśruta are considered as *vaidya* texts, they also give great importance for mantra:

ariṣṭāmapi mantraiśca badhnīyān mantrakovidaḥ /
sā tu rajjvādibhir baddhā viṣapratikarī matā //
devabrahmārṣibhiḥ proktā mantrāḥ satyatapomayāḥ /
bhavanti nānyathā kṣipraṃ viṣaṃ hanyuḥ sudustaram //
viṣaṃ tejomayair mantraiḥ satyabrahmatapomayaiḥ /
yathā nivāryate kṣipraṃ prayuktair na tathauṣadhaiḥ //
Suśruta 5.5:8-10 //
bhūtānāmadhipaṃ devaṃ Īśvaraṃ jagataḥ prabhum /
pūjayan prayato nityaṃ jayatyunmādajaṃ bhayam //
rudrasya pramathā nāma gaṇā loke caranti ye /
teṣāṃ pūjāṃ ca kurvāṇa unmādebhyaḥ pramucyate //
Caraka 6.9:91-92 //

Among the *tantra manuals* of Kerala, the *Īśānagurudeva-paddhati* could have been the first manual which treated 'toxicology' related matters. It describes about the different types of snakes (chapter 39), type of bites and how it affects a person, the inauspicious places to be bitten by a snake, parts of body where a snake bite could become serious, the signs of messenger who comes and informs the physician about a snake bite, the usage of mantras to destroy the reaction of poison, treatment for the bite of different types of snakes, treatment for the bite of scorpion, rat etc.

The *Tantrasārasaṅgraha* also deals with the similar topics on toxicology as dealt in the *Īśānagurudevapaddhati*. Śrī Brahmadattan Nambuthiri of Ullannoor Mana informs me that the methods prescribed in the *Tantrasārasaṅgraha* is extensively used in Kerala for snake bite treatment and many vernacular manuals in Kerala on this subject used the *Tantrasārasaṅgraha* as a source book. The second chapter of the *Tantrasārasaṅgraha* provides a detailed description of different types of snakes and snake bite, the sign of the messenger etc. The text describes the inauspicious places where snake-bite can occur:

> *devālaye śūnyagṛhe valmīkodyānakoṭare //*
> *rathyāsandhau caityatarau śmaśāne sindhusaṅgame /*
> *dvīpe catuṣpathe saudhe gahane vetrapadmayoḥ//*
> *parvatāgre biladvāre jīrṇakūpāśmakūṭayoḥ/*
> *śigruśleṣmātakākṣeṣu jambūdumbaraveṇuṣu//*
> *vaṭe 'tha jīrṇaprākāre daṃśaḥ sarpasya ninditaḥ /*
> 2:35cd-38ab

The third chapter of the *Tantrasārasaṅgraha* gives details of the treatment and also of the mantras to be used during the treatment. The divisions of poison, details of *vipattipañcākṣara, Gāruḍamantras* for the *viṣastambhana* etc. are dealt in this chapter. The fourth chapter provides the *Śaiva* mantras to be used for the treatment. The fifth and sixth chapter provides the details of different types of snake (brāmhaṇa etc.) and the treatment for snakebite. While the seventh chapter describes about the *gonasa* and *maṇḍali* snakes, the eighth chapter describes the snakes such as rājila. The ninth chapter is devoted to discuss different types of rat and the remedies for its poison. The tenth chapter describes the poison of spider and its treatments.

Thus the first ten chapters of the *Tantrasārasaṅgraha* is fully devoted to describe different types of poison treatment and hence this first ten chapters are very much practised even today for snake-bite treament.

The two unpublished manuals, the *Prayogasāra* (Ch. 37-40) and the *Yogaratnāvali* (Ch. 1) also deals with the treatment of different types of poisoning. *Prayogasāra* deals mostly on the treatment of poisoning, which include the symptoms of poison, detailed description of the *Garuḍamantra* etc. The thirty-eighth paṭala of *Prayogasāra* gives a detailed description of the *Garuḍamantra* and confirms that, with the usage of this mantra one could get rid of the *viṣa*—

sadyaḥ sarvātmanā śāntiṃ prayāti viṣamaṃ viṣam

The commentary *Sarvāṅgasundarī* by Vāsudeva on *Prayogasāra* elaborates many ideas mentioned in the text with many quotations, including the *Mantrasadbhāva, Mālinīvijaya, Uccuṣmabhairava, Sarvajñānottara* etc.

Health and Medicine in the Kerala Ritual Manuals

The Kerala manuals of *tantra* also contains descriptions related to the treatment of different type of diseases such as treatment for insane, treatment for different kinds of fevers, treatment for health related issues of children etc. It seems that the health of children was given importance, as we could see in the following verse of the *Īśānagurudevapaddhati*:

atha grahacikitsātra likhyate nātivistṛtā /
tatra bālacikitsāyāḥ prakārā bahudhā smṛtāḥ //
teṣvādau matamāśritya khaḍgarāvaṇacoditam /
nārāyaṇīyoditaṃ ca mārgadvayam ihocyate //
Īśānagurudevapaddhati 41:1-2 //

As we could see above, the *Khaḍgarāvaṇamantra* seems to be given great importance in most of the manuals dealing with treatments for illness and treatment for poisoning. The ninth chapter of *Kriyākālaguṇottara* gives full details of this mantra and we could see that the *Īśānagurudevapaddhati, Tantrasārasaṅgraha* and *Prayogasāra* follows it as prescribed in the *Kriyākālaguṇottara.*

Prayogasāra in its twenty-eighth chapter gives a detailed description of the reasons for infertility and its treatment:

atha santānasidhyartham pravakṣyāmi cikitsitam /
tatrādhāraṃ striyaḥ prāyas tāsu kāryā tataḥ kriyā //
daivadoṣagrahugrastāḥ striyo vandhyā bhavanti hi /
ṛtāvatau parīkṣyāstā vakṣyamāṇais tu lakṣaṇaiḥ // 28:1-2 //

And in its twenty-ninth chapter the methods for protecting the embryo and in thirtieth chapter the health issues related to new born and their remedies are discussed.

ataḥ paraṃ pravakṣyāmi garbharakṣāṃ samāsataḥ /
ādau guhasya rakṣārthaṃ devaiḥ sṛṣṭāḥ kila grahāḥ //29:1 //
ataḥ paraṃ pravakṣyāmi bālarakṣāṃ yathākramam /
prathame 'hani gṛhṇāti bālakaṃ pāvanīgrahī // 30:1 //

Conclusion

The above brief discussion on the 'systems of medicine' in the Kerala texts of *tantra* clearly makes us aware that the *tantra* texts were not only meant for rituals but were dealing with topics which are useful for one's day to day life. It is worth to note that, the two types of treatment, *viṣavaidya* (medicine) and *viṣavidyā* (*mantra*/medicine) are still followed in Kerala although *Viṣavidyā* is slowly disappearing.

Moreover, a survey of large manuscript catalogues reveals that hundreds of texts dealt with *Gāruḍa* and *Bhūtatantras*, as well as different systems of medicine, including toxicology. We currently have only a handful of non-critical editions of texts which may come under the group *Bhūtatantra* and *Gāruḍatantra*. Such important texts deserve critical editions, and the group as a whole deserve a survey and study. It is essential that the scientific reasons and metaphysical aspects hidden behind these ritual texts need to be explored and explained. But to enable to do this study, we require more texts on the topic since most of the ritual texts still remain in manuscript form.

NOTES

1. The text is reproduced here from the hand-out on *Kriyākālaguṇattara* provided by Dr. Michael J. Slouber during the First Early Tantra Workshop (2008) held at Kathmandu.
2. Some of the the important topics related to the systems of medicine that are dealt in the *Īśānagurudevapaddhati* (Vol. II): *Kevalarogaśānti* (p. 168), *Sarpajātibhedas tadutpatyādikramaśca* (p. 258), *Daṅśanabhedāḥ tallakṣaṇāni daṣṭasyāvasthāviśeṣāśca* (p. 260), *Aniṣṭasthānāni* (p. 262), *Dūtavākyākṣaraniyama* (p. 262), *Nimittāni* (p. 263), *Vipattimantrādhikāra* (p. 265), *Viṣaharaṇa-nānāmantradhyānaviniyogavidhāna* (p. 267), *Phaṇicikitsā* (p. 272), *Maṇḍalicikitsā* (p. 274), *Vṛścikacikitsā* (p. 278), *Ākhuviṣacikitsā* (p. 279), *Lūtacikitsā* (p. 281), *Nānā-prāṇiviṣacikitsā* (p. 282), *Khaḍgarāvaṇabālacikitsā* (p. 288), *Bālapīḍakagrahataceṣṭāḥ, tatpratikāravidhayaśca* (p. 292), *Grahāṇāṃ bhedāḥ, tadāviṣṭasya lakṣaṇaṃ, tadvimocanopāyśca* (p. 298), *Bhūtatantra* (p. 301), *Apasmāronmādacikitsādhikāra* (p. 311), *Nānārogacikitsādhikāra* (p. 331), *Āyurvardhanarasāyana* (p. 393), *Mṛtyuvijaya* (p. 394) etc.
3 The relationship between the *Īśānagurudevapaddhati* and the *Tantrasārasaṅgraha* are discussed in an article 'Khaḍga-Rāvaṇa and His worship in Balinese and Indian Tantric Sources', (in *Wiener Zeitschrift fur die Kunde Sudasiens,* 21, 1977, pp. 143-69) by Teun Goudriān.

BIBLIOGRAPHY

Īśānagurudevapaddhati of *Īśānaguru.* ed. T. Gaṇapati Śāstri, 4 Vols. Delhi: Bharatiya Vidya Prakashan, 1990. (Reprinted with a new introduction by N. P. Unāni, from Trivandrum Sanskrit Series Nos. 69, 72, 77 and 83. Trivandrum, 1920, 1921, 1922, 1925.)

Prayogasāra. Ms. 10307 of Oriental Research Institute and Ms. Library, Trivandrum.

Tantrasārasaṅgraha of Nārāyaṇa with the commentary Mantravimarśinī by Svarṇagrāma Vāsudeva. ed. N.V.P.

Unithiri. Calicut University Sanskrit Series 15 and 16, Publication Division, University of Calicut, 2002.

Yogaratnāvalī. Ms. T. 993, French Institute, Pondicherry.

"Khaḍga-Rāvaṇa and His worship in Balinese and Indian Tantric Sources," in *Wiener Zeitschrift fur die Kunde Sudasiens*, T. Goudriān, 1977, pp. 143–69.

13

Tamil Medical Manuscripts in the Oriental Research Institute and Manuscripts Library, Thiruvananthapuram

O. PADMAKUMARI

Our ancestors led a life intertwined with nature. This is known from their division of land into five classes with the names of plants: *Kurinji* (mountaneous region), *mullai* (forest region), *marutham* (cultivable region), *neital* (littoral region) and *palai* (desert region) based on their lifestyle. Plants became part and parcel of their life, since they lived with nature and they were quite familiar containing the medicinal qualities of the plants.

Treating the patients and saving their lives were noble deeds to them. Tamil medicine has the scientific heritage of more than 200 years. Hiding the medicines from others was considered to be a malicious sin. They preserved the names, preparation and the methods of medical treatment in palmleaf manuscripts. Most of the Tamil palm-leaf manuscripts are medical manuscripts with the traditional methods followed by the Tamils.

The *Keeltisai* Manuscripts Library of the Kerala University is the second greatest in Asia. More than 60,000 manuscripts are preserved here, among which, the Sanskrit and Malayalam manuscripts occupy the first and second places in number respectively. On the other hand, there are more than three thousand manuscripts in Tamil. They are on various subjects such as religion, medicine, praise, story, lyrics, legends, prophecy, astrology, justice, history of places, poetry (*kaviyam*), grammar, dictionary (*nikandu*), petite literature (*cittilakkiyam*), folk-song, drama, mantra, *rasavatam* (combination of metals, herbs and salt), mathematic, epics (*ithihasam*) and philosophy.

Among these, the medical manuscripts occupy the first place in number, and religious manuscripts the second. In ancient India two classes of medical methods existed. Ayurvedic medicine existed in the North and Siddha medicine in the South. Tamil medicine is the natural method of treating diseases, founded by the Tamils. The famous sage and poet Thiruvalluvar says in his *Thirukkural*:

His body needs no drugs who only eats
After digesting what he ate before. (942)

(If one takes proper food after digesting the food he already ate and when he feels hungry, the body won't be affected by any disease and no medicine will be needed.)

Tamil medicine is the one without any side effect. It lost its individuality by the impact of allopathy. Tamil medicine is preserved as a part of heritage in the countryside. Ancient history states that the pepper exported from Tamil Nadu is the Indian pain reliever with medicinal qualities.

In the Manuscript Library of Thiruvananthapuram, more than 125 manuscripts with the message on *rasavatham* and *kayakalpam* are found in Agathiyar's name. The manuscript *Agathia Nayanar Puranam* 150 explains stack storage and *Agathiyar Purana Soothiram* 216 gives the details of medicine, *mantra and attachithu*. In general, the manuscripts in Agathiyar's name comprise the details of medicinal names, preparation methods, symptoms of diseases and methods of curing them.

There are five manuscripts in the name of Romarishi, eight in Pinnakku Siddha's name, twelve in Poha Munivar's name, five in Idaikkadai Siddhar's name, seven in Ramadevar's name, ten in Konkanar's name, two in Kamala Muni's name, two in Karuvoor Siddhar's name, seven in Chattai Muni's name, three in Korakkar's name, eight in Nandhīśvarar's name, four in Thanvantari's name and three in Thirumoolar's name.

More than fifteen manuscripts on poison-treatment are there with details of *Poison treatment mantra yantirankal*, 'anti-venom of snakes' and 'chanting mantras'. Also many manuscripts on *Nāḍī Nidānam* and *Nāḍī Susthiram* (feeling the pulse) are there with precious message:

Anaitthuyiren tenni arumpasuyevarkkumūtri
Manatthulle pethāpetham vanchanai kalavum poiyum
Chinatthaiyum thavirppāyāhil cheithavam pin verundo
Unakkithu uruthiyāna vupathesa mithuve kandāi.

(If you get rid of your partiality, wickedness, stealth, lie and anger from your mind by thinking that all lives are precious, there will not be a great 'tavam' (meditation) than this. This is the strong catechism you have found).

The manuscript '*Nāḍī Nidānam*' reveals the astonishing truth that there are 4448 methods to diagnose the disease by feeling the pulse. The details of pulse is explained clearly in the manuscript 'Yukamuni Nāḍī'.

Nayanthu nee nādithān pārkkum pothu
Nalamāna puruva mucchi kandam nenchu
Kayanthu kaiyil kāladiyil muzhankai thannil
Kanakkālil muzhankālir kaikkuzhi yilāhum.

(While you feel the pulse, the diseases of eyebrows, head, body, chest, hands, legs, elbow, ankles and armpits can be found)

There are manuscripts on ophthalmology too. Four among them reveal *Nayanavīthi* treatment (treatment on the principle action of the eyes). From them, we know that there are 96 eye-diseases and the causes are rheumatic problems (45 diseases), *Silethma* (phlegm) problems (20 diseases), *pitta* (bile) problems (16 diseases) and 15 diseases in the eye muscles. The symptoms of these diseases and the treatment for them are given in simple methods.

More than twelve manuscripts on *Karpakkol* (pregnancy and conception) are available with the details of sterility and its treatment. *Agathiyar karpa soothiram* says:

ārappā ānmalade āhumallāl
Appane penmaladu yāthumillai.

(There is the possibility of a man to become impotent but it is impossible for a woman to become sterile.)

The manuscripts *Karpakkol* seems to be the revelation of reasons for sterility as a reply of a Chinese to the 'so called sterile women's prayer towards *Nemiyan* to recover from their sterility.

There are three manuscripts on the nature of diseases and types of medicines, more than fifteen on the medicine for various diseases, fifteen on the methods of medicine preparation, and eight manuscripts on *marunthu yokankal* (fortunate medicines). The manuscripts by name *Malayaharathi* (Mountain Dictionary) offers the names of medicines. Seven manuscripts under the title *Vaidyanighaṇṭu* (medicine dictionary), two under the title *Vaidya rathina surukkam* (a brief note on medicines), and six under the title *Agarathi Nighaṇṭu* (Dictionary of Dictionary) are also found.

Status of the Manuscripts

Form:

Manuscripts are mostly found in verse (*venpa*) form. It may be for memorizing and remembering easily. The manuscripts found in prosaic form are with colloquial words.

Time:

No information is found in the manuscripts about the time they were written.

Place:

A few manuscripts have the details of the author along with his native place. For example, in a manuscript, it is written as: Written by Subbuthevar, Son of Muthuthevar of Ramayan patti.

Author's name:

Some manuscripts are with the name of the authorized author.

e.g. *Agathiar Vaithiyan 1500*
Romarishi Gnana Soothiram.

Warnings:

Warning instructions such as: "If anyone takes this manuscript with evil intention, one will be affected with diseases like blindness, leprosy and other evils" are found in most of the manuscripts. From this, it can be assumed that some households of the ancient times functioned like today's libraries. Such warnings are mostly found in the medical manuscripts in order to avoid misusing them.

Conclusion

The Department is engaged in the task of preparing a Manuscript Explanatory Catalogue with the list of medical manuscripts in order to bring out the hidden treasure of Tamil medicine to the world. Arrangements are also made to transcribe the manuscripts and to publish them. Preventive measures to preserve the manuscripts are also taken. Through this, we can expect a revival of the Tamil hereditary medicine.

14

Textbook Tradition of Āyurveda

VINOD KUMAR

Āyurveda, the traditional health care system of India flourished approximately 2500 years back as a part of intellectual renaissance sustained at that time. The primitive man, after being satisfied with his instinctive and basic needs of life started observations and experimentations in the surroundings to make out principles behind the happenings around him. He started wondering on the diversity maintained in the nature and the character of his relation with his environment. Health care was one among central themes of his thoughts. Health has been conceived as something driven from outside, for which he symbolized super human forces to be the abodes of health. These forces, generally evils, entered his body to generate diseases, as believed; the treatment aimed at putting them out by means of prayers and even physical assaults. Along with prayers he started to use some herbs which he found effective through constant observations over animals.The *Atharvaveda,* which includes some amount of the system of sorcery and witch-crafting mainly addressed the problem of health hazards. Internal use of herbs made tremendous advance in the direction of phyto-pharmacological identification of the flora. In that way, the *Atharvaveda* paved way to different experimentations regarding the pharmacological actions of plans in a living system. The pre-vedic evidences of Indus

Valley Civilization excavated from Mahanjadaro suggested high quality of health care prevailing at that period.

It was towards the end of Vedic period (2200–1000 BC), India entered the new era of intellectual renaissance through the emergence of philosophical thoughts (*darśanas*). The analytical methodology implemented by philosophical thought influenced the health care practices at that time. The masters, with the help of powerful philosophical inputs, tried to build a theoretical platform for the medical practice then existed. Thus, the emergence of Āyurveda established the evolution of scientific material based on experimentations. When philosophy stood as mere intellectual exercises, applied sciences like Āyurveda tried to translate them to the need of common man. Instead of tracking to the restricted outlook of individual philosophies, Āyurveda tried to adopt the philosophical thoughts from different philosophies in whatever manner they become beneficial to mankind. Naturally, it came that, Āyurveda did not blindly follow any particular philosophy, but, made use of the philosophies as raw materials to build its own scientific material. No wonder that Āyurveda took the privilege to manipulate the philosophical inputs, solely for the betterment of mankind.

Vedas–the early footprints

The earliest written document of medical practice available hail from the Vedic literature, especially the *Atharvaveda*. The great masters of Āyurveda, Suśruta and Caraka consider the *Atharvaveda* as the sprouting land of Āyurveda.[1] Kāśyapa, a master in paediatrics, points out that the origin of Āyurveda is from Upanishads also. The *Atharvaveda* profoundly explains early, and definitely primitive and tribal, medical practices in the forms of *mantra*, sacrifices etc. The *Atharvaveda* described names related to diseases, anatomical description of human body, disease causing germs (commonly called as *kṛmi*), methods for their eradication, healing power of sun-rays, medicinal qualities of water and air, some surgical procedures for treatment of urinary calculus and medicinal use of over 200 herbs.

In Ṛgveda, the chief descriptions were regarding the wonder treatments done by divine personalities like Aśvin-twins in various diseases of divine and earthly persons. The mantras in the form of prayers to Aśvin twins were chanted to achieve longevity, health and drugs for treating various ailments. Description of different kinds of poisons, germs and many diseases are available in the *Ṛgveda*. In *Yajurveda*, especially *Śuklayajurveda*, description of curative qualities of drugs, alleviation of diseases like *arśas* (piles), *śvayathu* (edema), *ślīpada* (filariasis) etc., anatomy of horses and human beings are available.The *Sāmaveda* contains many hymns apart from those in the *Ṛgveda*.

The main difference of approach to medical care in the *Atharvaveda* and the *Ṛgveda* was that the former tried to heal the ailment through various procedures and application of medicines, the latter through the result of divine powers which were not subjected to practical analysis. The *Atharvaveda* used practical ways of treatment, but the *Ṛgveda* tried to invoke divine personalities to get a cure from the diseases. This vividly explains the priority in influence of the *Atharvaveda* on Āyurveda; because, Āyurveda definitely took the way of practical application.

Traditions – Pan-Indian and regional

The formation and development of Ayurvedic textbook tradition could be traced to chiefly in two distinct tracks. One is a pan-Indian, Sanskrit dominant tradition and the other is regional traditions prevailed at different geographical areas, mostly non-Sanskrit. These two parallel traditions differ by way of many critical factors. (see table 1a)

Table 1a. Comparison between Pan-Indian and Regional

traditions

Pan Indian tradition		Regional tradition
Language	Sanskrit language	Mostly regional
Content	Containing all branches branches	Mostly any one of the
Authorship	Claimed by an author authorship	Mostly anonymous
Orientation	Theory oriented	Practical oriented
Structure	Well structured with sections, chapters etc.	Not necessarily well structured
Influence of philosophies	Well identified	Not identified
Availability	Available anywhere concealed in familial	Local availability or traditions
Learning	As a part of formal Sanskrit tradition,	Mostly informal learning in families especially Gurukula

SAṂHITĀKĀLA—THE CLASSICAL AGE OF TEXTUAL TRADITION

With the strong theoretical support imparted by philosophies, the masters of Āyurveda tried to evolve with the theoretical foundation during the *saṃhitā* period (500 BC–600 AD) with the emergence of major textbooks called *saṃhitās*. It was during this period that the traditional medical system was designated as Āyurveda. The initial phase of this period was 'phase of specialization', that means, different specialties were practised by masters of those particular fields. For example, paediatricians, surgeons, toxicologists etc. But, the scenario changed by the end of the *saṃhitā* period. There came the idea of comprehensive medicine which tried to incorporate all the branches under one resort. This change was obviously visible in the making of different textbooks also. During this period the knowledge base of Āyurveda got many revisions so that the scientific content flourished under different domains separately. Mainly eight branches came into existence. Even then, the most popular branches remained as General Medicine (*kāyacikitsā*) and Surgery (*Śalyacikitsā*), which found themselves as complementary to each other. Other branches also got represented by different masters and textbooks (see table-1b). Among these textbooks, three major compendia namely *Carakasaṃhitā*, *Suśrutasaṃhitā* and the *Aṣṭāṅgasaṅgraha* got a separate superior status among textbooks and became popular as Major triad (*bṛhattrayī*). The important features of *bṛhattrayī* can be summarized as follows:

1. They paved the strong theoretical foundation to Āyurveda
2. They tried to represent all the eight branches of Āyurveda under one resort
3. They contained all practical aspects of Āyurveda including diagnosis, therapeutics, pharmacology, pharmacy, different procedures, outcomes of treatment, etc.
4. They represented the paradigm shift from pure philosophy to practical philosophy.

Table – 1b. Main textbooks in the Saṃhitākāla

Sl. No.	Name of textbook	Author	Speciality	Approximate period
1	Kāśyapasaṃhitā	Vṛddhajīvaka	Paediatrics (bālacikitsā)	6th Century BC
2	Suśrutasaṃhitā	Suśruta	Surgery, anatomy	4th Century BC
3	Carakasaṃhitā	Caraka	General medicine (kayacikitsā)	1st Century AD
4	Aṣṭāngasaṅgraha	Vāgbhaṭa, the senior	All branches	4th Century AD
5	Aśṭāṅgahṛdaya (concised edition of Aṣṭāṅgasaṅgraha)	Vāgbhaṭa, the junior	All branches	6th Century AD

Saṃhitā–product of many masters

Textbooks of the Saṃhitā period generally and strongly adhered to specific patterns of teaching and learning which prevailed at that period. Textbooks got documented in palm manuscripts written on palmleaves, birchbarks, etc. after being repeatedly modified through a methodology which emphasized on learning through memorizing and chanting the material, especially in the presence and guidance of masters. Naturally textbooks were written as reports of discussion between the master and his disciples regarding different topics. The master or adviser makes authentic comments where disciples got ample opportunities to interact with him. Some instances show that there were discussions with other masters, called *tadvidyasambhāṣā,* regarding some topics to rectify the incongruity regarding those topics. The style of presentation of scientific material in *Carakasaṃhitā* and *Suśrutasaṃhitā* supports the above view. These texts contain four types of verses (*sūtras*).[2] They are:

1. Those advised by the master (*gurusūtra*)
2. Those in the form of queries by the disciple (*Śiṣyasūtra*)
3. Those added by the redactor later as a part of updating the science (*pratisaṃskartṛsūtra*)
4. Those proposed by disciples as a part of discussion which later gets settled by the master (*ekīyasūtra*)

The master, often referred to as the adviser (*upadeṣṭā*), was regarded as founder of the specialty dealt in the textbook. In *Carakasaṃhitā,* the adviser was Ātreya, who was considered to be the founder of Medical tradition, customarily known as Ātreya tradition. On the other hand, in *Suśrutsaṃhitā,* the advisor was Dhanvantari, the founder of surgical tradition. In paediatrics, the tradition was founded by Kāśyapa, the advisor of the *Kāśyapasaṃhitā.* The author of the textbook (*granthakartā*) in each tradition was the disciple of the master. Where there was more than one disciple for the same master, all of them wrote their own textbooks, with great variability in popularity. With a few exceptions, almost all the textbooks were named after the corresponding authors. Naturally they showed considerable resemblance regarding structure and content. Many of them were lost partially or completely afterwards. (please see the title—'lost textbooks')

Almost all the major textbooks were subjected to major redactions in a later period. A redactor (*pratisaṃskartā*) renewed the textbook by updating it through summarizing over explained areas and elaborating areas which needed to.[3] Redactors made major changes in the content of *Carakasaṃhitā* and the *Suśrutsaṃhitā*. In the case of *Carakasaṃhitā*, the original textbook written by *Agniveśu*, disciple of Ātreya, wrote his own textbook namely *Agniveśa-saṃhitā*, which was later redacted by Caraka, later became famous as *Carakasaṃhitā*. In third century AD, Dṛḍhabala made second redaction to the textbook, with major changes. He added forty-one chapters to the textbook, including two sections. In the case of the *Suśrutasaṃhitā*, the redaction was done by Nāgārjuna (second century AD), who completed the textbook by adding the whole second part (Uttaratantra) of the textbook containing 66 chapters. The *Kāśyapasaṃhitā*, after being lost for a long period was recovered by Vātsya, who made redaction in matter and style. In the *Aṣṭāṅgasangrahu*, the latest of greater triad (fourth century AD), the author (Vāgbhaṭa, the senior) claims that the textbook itself is updated according to the need of time (*yugānurūpa-sandarbha*). It was within two centuries of its creation, Vāgbhaṭā, the junior (sixth century AD) published its concised edition, *Aṣṭāṅgahṛdaya*, with necessary modifications and updating. In fact, this edition served the purpose of redaction in a better manner. Moreover, the *Aṣṭāṅgahṛdaya* marked the end of the golden age of the Saṃhitā periodof *Āyurveda.*

Saṃhitā tradition: some facts

The Saṃhitā tradition of Āyurveda marked the major shift from mystic character of health care practices to empirical forms. The former was sustained through tribal and folk based know-hows regarding healing properties of plants. But, in the *Saṃhitās*, the same practices got firm theoretical foundations. Through this change, the scientific and structured study and practice of Āyurveda became a part of the so called 'noble tradition' sustained through the discourse of Sanskrit. Since then, there existed two distinct parallel streams of traditions: the tribal and the noble. Most of the textbooks written in Sanskrit thus became assets of the noble tradition. Then also some masters put hints in their textbooks to admit that tribal contributions were not negligible in the study regarding plants. A change in this structure occurred due to the influence of the Buddhism and Jainism in health care practices. Institutionalization of medical practice was the major change installed by Buddhist tradition. Later masters like Vāgbhaṭa were greatly influenced by Buddhism, evidently visible in his textbook, Aṣṭāṅgahṛdaya.

The socio-cultural standards prevailed at that period made serious impacts on the scientific content of the *Saṃhitās*. Beliefs, morals, values and code of conducts of the society became influential not only to the scientific content but also to the mode of presentation of the textbooks. Description of mythological stories/characters are found to be augmenting the credibility of the textbooks. Masters added serious philosophical discussions (beyond all their practical implications) in the textbooks to satisfy intellectuals. Religious practices also got ample allocations to make it digestive to people at large. Beyond all these ornamentations, the masters laid the golden threads of scientific spirit, throughout the whole content of their textbooks. So, a scholar, who approaches seriously and critically to analyze the *Saṃhitās*, should try to distinguish mythological, historical, philosophical and scientific content in them.

Śāstra and Tantra

In ancient India, any systematic knowledge was known as *Śāsstra*. *Śāstra* was that which commands or teaches (*Śāsana*) some instructions related to different spheres of life. Moral preachings (*Nītiśāstra*), instructions of law (*Dharmaśāstra*), commercial and administrative rules (*Arthaśāstra*), philosophical thoughts (*Darśanaśāstra*), erotic compositions (*Kāmaśāstra*), etc. were the famous *śāstras* of that time. In that way Āyurveda also is a *śāstra*. Terms like *śākhā, tantra, vidyā, sūtra, lakṣaṇa, jñāna,* etc. also were used as synonyms of *śāstra* as far as Āyurveda was concerned.[4] In a closer observation it is vividly understood that these synonyms meet the scopes of different discourses of science, that is,

1. Science in toto—*śāstra, vidyā, jñāna*
2. A specific branch of that science—*śākhā*
3. Technological aspect of the science—*tantra*
4. Literature of a particular science—*sūtra*
5. Technical terminologies of the science –*lakṣaṇa*

Then also, terms used most frequently to denote 'textbook' are *śāstra* and *tantra.*

Features of ideal science/textbook

A person who wants to learn a particular *śāstra* should examine it considering the ideal qualities designed for a *śāstra.* Those qualities are related to the genuineness of the science as well as the credibility of the textbooks.[5]

1. Certified by experts (*sumahad-yasasvi-dhīrapuruṣā-sevita*)
2. Rich in content (*arthabahula*)
3. Followed by authentic scholars (*āptajanapūjita*)
4. Palatable to pupils of different intellectual capacity (*trividhaśiṣyabuddhihita*)
5. Devoid of repetition (*apagatapunaruktadoṣa*)
6. Well explained aphorisms, explanations and compila-

tions (*supraṇītasūtrabhāṣyasaṅgrahakrama*)

7. Self-explanatory (*svādhāra*)
8. Devoid of colloquial usage of language (*anavapatitaśabda*)
9. Devoid of complicated terms (*akaṣṭāśabda*)
10. Use of non-fabricated language (*puṣkalābhidhāna*)
11. Sequential explanation of technical terms (*kramāgatārtha*)
12. Giving importance to illustrate technical terms (*arthatattvaviniścayapradhāna*)
13. Explaining relevant theories only (*saṅgatārtha*)
14. Devoid of jumbling different sub-topics (*asaṅkulaprakaraṇa*)
15. Rich in definitions (*lakṣaṇavat*)
16. Rich in illustrative examples (*udāharaṇavat*)

There are fifteen defects (*tantradoṣa*) by which a textbook becomes worthless for learning. They are:[6]

1. Use of uncommon words (*aprasiddhaśabda*)
2. Use of wrong interpretations (*duṣpraṇīta*)
3. Use of words with difficult pronunciation (*asukhārohipada*)
4. Irrelevant descriptions (*asaṅgatārtha*)
5. Statements contradicted by its illustration (*viruddha*)
6. Over-explained principles (*ativistṛta*)
7. Over-summarized principles (*atisamkṣipta*)
8. Doubtful descriptions (*sandigdha*)
9. Repetitions (*punarukta*)
10. Descriptions without proper references (*niṣpramāṇa*)
11. Descriptions without proper objective (*niṣprayojana*)
12. Non-completion of statements (*asamāptākṣara*)
13. Statement contradictory to previously established principle (*vyāhṛta*)
14. Meaningless statements (*apārthaka*)
15. Disordered description (*bhinnakrama*)

Content and structure of saṃhitās

Almost all textbooks in the *saṃhita* period tried to incorporate the description regarding all the eight branches then existed in Āyurveda. The preference given to different branches varied. (See table-1). The branches are, general medicine (*kāyacikitsā*), paediatrics (*bālacikitsā or kaumārabhāṣya*), psychiatry (*grahacikitsā* or *bhūtavidyā*), ENT/ophthalmology (*śālākyatantra*), surgery (*śalyatantra*), toxicology (*daṃṣtrā-cikitsā* or *agadatantra*), rejuvenative therapy (*jarācikitsā* or *rasāyana*) and reproductive medicine (*vajikaraṇatantra*). Description of basic principles (*siddhānta*), preventive medicine (*svasthavṛtta*), pharmacology (*dravyaguṇa*), pharmacy (*bhaiṣajyakalpana*) and therapeutic procedures (*kriyākrama*) are common to all branches, and are described separately.

The whole content of the textbooks are divided into different sections (*sthāna*). Each section deals with a specific aspect of the science. Sections contain different chapters, the name of which explains its contents. Chapters will discuss principles under different contexts (*prakaraṇa*). Each context contains many aphorisms (*sūtra*) or verses (*śloka*) to explain the proposed concept. The main sections seen in an Ayurvedic textbook are:

1. *Sūtrasthāna*—dealing mainly with basic principles and preventive medicine
2. *Śārīrasthāna*—embryology, anatomy and physiology
3. *Nidānasthāna*—pathology
4. *Kalpasthāna*—pharmacy and therapeutic procedures
5. *Cikitsāsthāna*—treatment
6. *Uttarasthāna*—appendix part for remaining branches

Vāgbhaṭa firmly followed the above structure while making his textbooks. In that way his textbooks (*Aṣṭāṅgahṛdaya* and *Aṣṭāṅgasaṅgraha*) are considered to be the most structured ones among all the textbooks written so far. Other textbooks show slight misappropriations in allocating chapters to different sections. Some of them contained more sections also (Vimānasthāna, Siddhisthāna and Indriyasthāna in the *Carakasaṃhitā;* Khilasthāna in the *Kāśyapasaṃhitā*). In fact, those textbooks, having more sections, imparted extensive descriptions, sometimes irrelevant for a beginner. Later, Vāgbhaṭa omitted those sections by reallocating the content to one or other of the above sections. This reductionistic approach helped to make the content highly precise and definitive so that the scholars found it easy to learn Āyurveda. Even then, the higher texts like the *Carakasaṃhitā* and *Suśrutasaṃhitā* became helpful in attaining deeper knowledge about specific topics. Putting in other words, Vāgbhaṭa's textbooks, especially the *Aṣṭāṅgahṛdaya* is the learner's manual and the higher texts like the *Carakasaṃhitā* and the *Suśrutasaṃhitā* are the researcher's manuals.

Style and Language

Majority of classical Ayurvedic literature are credited to the Sanskrit language. Traditional textbooks available in regional languages including Malayalam and Tamil documented many of the regional specialties in practices. All the textbooks of greater triad were stylized as blend of ślokas and prose. But the *Aṣṭāṅgahṛdaya* and later texts of the *saṅgraha* period used *ślokas* only to represent scientific material. Rare textbooks like the *Rasavaiśeṣikasūtra* (written by Bhadanta Nāgārjuna) followed aphorism (*sūtra)* style of literature. *Sūtras* always needed sufficient commentaries for proper understanding. It is not accidental in a practical science like Āyurveda that the scientific material did not get presented in a more complicated style of *sūtra,* which always needs experts' assistance to get the meanings. In regional practices like that in Kerala, the common trend was to document the knowledge in regional languages, with few exceptions like the *Ārogyakalpadruma* (written by

Kaikkulangara Rama Varier), a regional text in paediatrics from Kerala.

Techniques of decoding textbooks–Tantrayukti

Another peculiarity of these textbooks was use of *tantrayukti* for their correct composing and interpretation. Unlike other forms of literature, the technical language and presentation have many limitations. Scope of imagination should be kept minimum in scientific textbooks; where, other forms of literature like kāvya etc. can have it at any range. *Tantrayukti* helps to bring uniform interpretations of a textbook by different persons at different point of time. Use of *tantrayukti* brings appropriation of sense and sentences (*vākyayojana* and *arthayojana*). *Arthaśāstra* and *saṃhitās* in Āyurveda use *tantrayuktis* as codes for scientific interpretation.

MEDIEVAL PERIOD—THE AGE OF COMPILATIONS

The classical age was followed by the age of compilations (*saṅgrahakāla,* 7th Century–17th century AD), customarily called medieval period (*mādhyamika kāla*). This period marked the end of original and innovative thoughts in the science, but, sustained the reflected glory of the classical age. Because, almost all the treatises created in this period showed greater affinity to the content of classical texts. These textbooks customarily called 'compilations' (*saṅgrahagrantha*) were specialized in any one of different scopes of Āyurveda, purely accepting the classical texts as foundation. In that way these texts made an opportunity for the advancement of individual subjects. This period, otherwise called 'transitional age', witnessed to major transitions in dynasties and to the interactions with other systems of medicines like Unani, Tibb and Chinese medicines at different points of times. The advancements mainly happened in pathology (*nidāna*), pharmacy (*bhaiṣajyakalpana*), pharmacology (*dravyaguṇavijñāna*), therapeutics (*cikitsā*) and allied disciplines like alchemy (*rasaśāstra*), traditional veterinary medicine (*mṛgāyurveda*), Āyurveda for plants (*vṛkṣāyurveda*) and *siddha* system. The inter relations with other countries resulted in arrival of new diseases, new diagnostic methods, new medicines, new pharmaceutical formulations, etc. Thus, it became a necessity to add appendices to classical texts in the above aspects, but, it happened in the form of creation of new textbooks specialized in those specific areas. These textbooks were not independent or self sufficient, because, every time the readers need to rely on the classical texts for deeper and essential understanding of principles. They only added the new developments to the list existed in classical texts. So, major content of those textbooks happened to be the compilation of the information available in classical texts, with minor modifications. Either they copied the verses from the classical texts or expressed the same idea in a different dictum. Development of *rasasāstra* and *siddha* medicines contributed a lot to the field of pharmacy including distillation, methods of fermentation, advancements in the making of tablets (*gulika*), and use of advanced equipments.

In the light of the above transition, textbooks written in this period fell in the following categories:

1. Textbooks of pathology and diagnostics (*roganidāna*)
2. Textbooks of Pharmacy (*bhaiṣajyakalpana*)
3. Textbooks of pharmacology (*dravyaguṇavijñāna*) and Lexicons (*nighaṇṭu*)
4. Major commentaries of classic texts
5. Textbooks of *rasaśāstra*
6. Textbooks for treatment (*cikitsāgraṅtha*)
7. Pharmacopoea (*yogagrantha*)
8. Textbooks related to traditional veterinary medicine and plant medicine

The minor triad–(laghutrayī)

Three textbooks, one each on diagnostics, pharmacy and pharmacology, were marked as the face-books broadcast ing the major trends of changes in medieval period (see table-2). They are popularly known as minor triad (*laghutrayī*) and considered to be the masterpieces in the subjects concerned. They added substantially to the respective content of classical texts, by incorporating new information regarding their topics. New diseases were explained in *Mādhavanidāna*, new processes in *Śārṅgadharasaṃhitā* and new drugs in the *Bhāvaprakāśa*. Chronologically they marked the whole medieval period at three intervals of four centuries each.

Table – 2. Minor triad (*laghutrayī*)

Sl. No.	Name of textbook	Author	Specialty	Approximate period
1	Mādhavanidāna	Mādhavakara or Rugviniścaya	Pathology and diagnostics (nidāna)	7th-8th century AD
2	Śārṅgadharasaṃhitā	Śārṅgadhara	Pharmacy (bhaiṣajya-kalpana)	12th -13th century AD
3	Bhāvaprakāśa	Bhāvamiśra	Pharmacology (dravyaguṇa-vijñāna)	17th century AD

Lexicons (nighaṇṭu)

Lexicons are the most valuable contribution of medieval period. They are textbooks where drugs (plants, animal products or minerals) are classified based on their pharmacological properties and their pharmacological/ botanical properties are summarized with maximum precision. In classical texts, the drugs were explained mainly as drug-groups (*auṣadhagaṇas*) or drug-recipes (*auṣadha-yoga*). Naturally, the therapeutic properties of such groups/

recipes goes to the clustered effect of all the ingredients in that group. There it was very difficult to know properties of individual drugs. In fact, classical texts also contained verses describing individual properties of different materials, especially food ingredients, but, they were insufficient in explaining majority of drugs. Moreover, it became an essentiality for practitioners to know the properties of individual drugs to conveniently prepare new formulations where classical texts failed to furnish sufficient guidelines.

Lexicons put a new trend by giving individual description of plants and other materials having medicinal importance. Description of individual plants includes their synonyms, pharmacological properties and sometimes therapeutic usages. A primitive style of lexicon is available in the *Amarakośa*, where names of plants and their synonyms are enlisted for reference. In lexicons, plants were classified based on some pharmacological features, and all the drugs in such groups were explained individually. In that way, lexicons served as ready-reckoners of practitioners in their daily practice. Single drug remedies also became popular. Some later lexicons added new drugs imported from abroad and some others identified substitutes for plants which were endangered or rare. In that way, lexicons became the most updated sources of pharmacology. Most of the lexicons were written as independent treatises, but, some like *Bhāvaprakāśanighaṇṭu* were written as an appendix to the textbook in the same name. Generally lexicons enlisted the drugs used in treatments of diseases irrespective of speciality. Some lexicons dealt with do's and dont's (*pathyāpathya*) related to treatments also. (see table-3). Putting in nutshell, a physician became handicapped in the absence of lexicons.

Table—3. Important Lexicons (*nighaṇṭus*)

Sl. No.	Name of textbook	Author	Approximate period
1	Dhanvantarinighṇṭu	Dhanvantari	Before 5 AD
2	Aṣṭāṅganighaṇṭu	Vāgbhaṭa	8th century AD
3	Siddhasāranighaṇṭu	Ravigupta	
4	Madanapālanighaṇṭu (*Madanavinoda*)	Madanapāla	13th century AD
5	Kaiyadevanighaṇṭu (*Pathyāpathyavibodhaka*)	Kaiyadeva	14th century AD
6	Rājanighaṇṭu (*Abhidhānacūdamaṇi*)	Narahari	14th century AD
7	Bhāvaprakāśanighaṇṭu	Bhāvamiśra	17th century AD
8	Nighaṇṭuratnākara	Vasudev Godbole	18th century AD
9	Śaligrāmanighaṇṭu	Śāligrāmavaidya	18th century AD
10	Nighaṇṭu Adarsh	Vaidya Bapalal	19th century AD
11	Auṣadhanighaṇṭu (Malayalam)	Thayyil Kumarakṛṣṇan	19th century AD

Textbooks on Rasaśāstra

Another major feature of the medieval period was development in the field of internal use of metals and minerals, called Rasaśāstra. This system developed in continuation to the advancement in the field of alchemy. Even though the classical textbooks mention the internal use of metals and minerals, they were secondary to that of herbal medicines. It was in medieval period that this branch flourished separately as an independent system. The literature in this system mainly focused on sources and availability of metals and minerals and different processes for making metals and minerals suitable for internal use. Nāgārjuna was considered to be the master of Rasaśāstra. Siddha system of medicine shows high resemblance with principle and practice of Rasaśāstra. The *Rasaratnasamucaya* (11th century AD) written by Vāgbhaṭa is considered as the most authentic textbook in Rasaśāstra. Important scientific descriptions like flame test of metals, complications of intake of toxic metals; antidotes of toxic metals, etc. are richly available in the text books of Rasaśāstra. See table (table-4) for details of the textbooks.

Table –4: Important textbooks on *Rasaśāstra*

Sl. No.	Name of textbook	Author	Approximate period
1	Rasaratnasamucchaya	Vāgbhaṭa	11th century AD
2	Rasaratnākara	Nāgārjuna	5th century AD
3	Rasakakṣaputa	Nāgārjuna	5th century AD
4	Rasārṇava	Unknown	12th century AD
5	Rasendracūdāmaṇi	Somadeva	12th century AD
6	Rasaprakāśasudhākara	Yeśodhara	13th century AD
7	Rasendrasārasaṅgraha	Gopāl a Bhaṭṭa	13th centrury AD
8	Rasajalanidhi	Bhudev Mukherji	19th century AD

Commentaries on classic texts

The most valuable commentaries on all *saṃhitās* were written in medieval period. The commentators made enormous contributions to the correct understanding of the *saṃhitās*. Commentators, flowrishing a later point of time, made critical comments on the *saṃhitās* with a comparative assessment of different authors. It was from the commentaries that later scholars came to know about the wealth of textual tradition sustained in Āyurveda, which were lost afterwards (see the topic lost textbooks). Some commentators wrote commentaries on more than one texts, exceptionally for all of the major triad (Jejjaṭa). There are many commentaries on one text, varying in nature and content, at different points of time. The textbooks in medieval period also got valuable commentaries on a later period. (See table-5)

Table–5. Important commentaries of major textbooks

Sl. No.	Name of textbook	Name of commentary	Name of commentator	Approximate period
1	Carakasaṃhitā	Āyurvedadīpikā	Cakrapāṇidatta	13th century AD
2	Suśrutasaṃhitā	Nibandhasaṅgraha	Ḍalhaṇa	10th century AD
3	Aṣṭāngasaṅgraha	Śaśīleka	Indu	13th century AD
4	Aṣṭāṅgahṛdaya	Sarvāṅgasundara	Arunadatta	13th century AD
5	Mādhavanidāna	Madhukoṣa	Śrīksnṭhadatta, Vijayarakshita	13th century AD
6	Śārṅgadhara-saṃhitā	Dīpikā	Āḍhamalla	15th century AD

Textbooks on allied disciplines

The mediaval age witnessed to sprouting and development of medicine for animals and plants. From the vedic period itself, people were familiar with those practices informally. Increased incidence of wars necessitated separate systems for animal care, especially horses and elephants. Rare references in classical texts described diseases affecting animals and therapeutic procedures applied in them. It was later in the medieval period that hastyāyurveda/aśvāyurveda/gavāyurveda developed with advancements. Textbooks like *Pālakāpya, Mātaṅgalīlā*, etc., are considered as masterpiece of elephant medicine. Salihotra, Bhoja, Nakula and Jayadatta were masters of horse medicine.

Vṛkṣāyurveda, medicine for plants, developed separately with specific formulations and methodologies. The '*Śārṅgadharapaddhati*' is considered as the authentic textbook of Vṛkṣāyurveda. (see table–6)

Table-6. Textbooks on allied sciences

Sl. No.	Name of textbook	Author	Specialty
1.	Pālakāpyam	Pālakāpya	Elephant medicine
2.	Mātaṅgalīlā		Elephant medicine
3.	Śālihotram	Śālihotra	Horse medicine
4.	Śyainakaśāstra	Rudradeva	Bird medicine
5.	Śārṅgadharapaddhati	Śārṅgadhara	Plant medicine

and Other text books and authors in medieval

Name	Author	Period Cent.	Content
Yogataraṅgiṇī	Thrimallabhatta	17 AD	General treatment
Dravyaguṇaśataka	Thrimallabhatta	17 AD	Pharmacology
Āyurvedasaukhya	Todarmal	16 AD	
Siddhayoga	Vṛnda	9 AD	General treatment
Cikitsākalikā	Tīsata	10 AD	General treatment
Cikitsāsaṅgraha (Cakradatta)	Cakrapāṇidatta	13 AD	General treatment
Dravyaguṇasaṅgraha	Cakrapāṇidatta	13 AD	Pharmacology
Paryāyaratnamālā	Mādhava	10 AD	Pharmacology
Yogasaṅgraha	Vṛndamādhava	9 AD	Pharmacopoea
Cikitsāsārasaṅgraha	Vaṅgasena	13 AD	Treatment
Yogaratnākara	Unknown	16 AD	Treatment
Bhaiṣajyaratnāvali	Govindadāsa	18 AD	Treatment
Ātaṅkatimirabhāṣya	Vaidya Balaram	18 AD	Treatment
Yogaratnasamuccaya	Candraṭa	10 AD	Pharmacopoea
Gadanigraha	Soḍhala	12 AD	Pharmacopoea
Guṇasaṅgraha	Soḍhala	12 AD	Lexicon
Śataślokī	Vopadeva	13 AD	Pharmacopoea
Bāsavarājīyam	Bāsavarāj	15 AD	Pharmacopoea
Yogacintāmaṇi	Harṣakīrti	17 AD	Pharmacopoea
Vaidyamanoramā	Kālidasa	19 AD	Pharmacopoea
Siddhabheṣajamaṇimālā	Kṛṣṇarāma-bhaṭṭa	19 AD	Pharmacopoea
Vaidyajīvana	Lolimbarāja	16 AD	Vaidyak kavya
Pathyāpathyaviniścaya	Viswanatha Sen	18 AD	Yunani
Pathyāpathya	Hikmath Prakash Mahadev		

KERALA'S CONTRIBUTION TO AYURVEDIC LITERATURE

Ayurvedic Textbooks written in Kerala itself broadcast the wealth of the tradition sustained here through centuries. These textbooks need not be counted as contribution of a person (author) but collective contribution of tradition as such. Most of the textbooks are anonymous in authorship and found to be edited and supplemented through different generations. Palm leaf manuscripts thus written were seen concealed in traditional families for many years. The language used in majority of textbooks is Manipravālam (combination of Malayalam and Sanskrit) and rarely Sanskrit. Some of the texts show vivid influence of Siddha system of medicine and they are written in Tamil—Malayalam combination. Most of the textbooks are practicality oriented; the theoretical descriptions if any, are taken from classic texts like the *Aṣṭāṅgahṛdaya*. The first available medical treatise in Kerala is thought to be *Alathūr manipravālam,* the manuscript of which is retrieved recently from Trissur Taikkat family and published by Kottakkal Āryavaidyaśālā. Later texts like *Cikitsāmañjari* and *Yagāmṛtam* show resemblance with this text. It was later in 18th century, the textbooks in Kerala was found with an obvious authorship. Before that, the textbooks were transferred through traditional families, anonymous in authorship. The *Rasavaiśeṣikasūtra,* written by Bhadanta Nāgārjuna is believed to be of Kerala origin, which traverses a different track in content and language. Apart from other textbooks, the same work deals with pure theoretical discussions, that too in Sanskrit, again in *sūtra* style of presentation. Generally, Kerala traditional textbooks deal with toxicology, general treatment, paediatrics and marmacikitsā. Some of them are mere collections of medicinal recipes (*yogagrantha*). Later, in 19th century, some textbooks written in Sanskrit dealt with modern anatomy and physiology. (see table–7)

Apart from the above, many valuable commentaries of *Aṣṭāṅgahṛdaya* were written by Keralites. Some examples are, *Sārārthadarpaṇa* by Kaikkulangara Ramavarier, *Bhāskara-*

vyākhyāna by Uppottu Kannan, *Aruṇodayam* by Govindan Vaidyar and *Hṛdayabodhikā* by Śrīdāsa Pandita. Some masters opine that famous commentator of the Aṣṭāṅgasaṅgraha, Indu was a Keralite.

Table–7. Textbooks of Kerala origin

Sl. No.	Name of Text	Author	Content	Language
1	Rasavaiseṣikasūtra	Bhadanta Nagarjuna	Basic Principles of Āyurveda	Sanskrit
2	Alathūr manipravalam	Unknown (a person from alathoor family)	General treatment	Manipravalam
3	Cikitsāmañjarī	Unknown	General treatment	,,
4	Sahasrayoga	Unknown	Compilation of drug formulations for different diseases	,,
5	Yogāmṛta	Unknown	Compilation of drug formulations for different diseases	,,
6	Vaidyatāraka	C.N. Narayanan	Pediatrics	Malayalam
7	Vaidyamanoramā	Unknown	Practical treatment of diseases	Sanskrit
8	Dhārākalpa	Unknown	Procedures of Pañcakarma	Sasnkrit
9	Sindūramañjarī	Thrissour thaikkattu Narayanan Mūsś	Rasaśāstra (medicinal application of metals and minerals)	
10	Cikitsanūl	General treatment	Manipravāla	
11	Āyurveda Auṣadha Nighaṇṭu	Thayyil Kumara Krishna description of drugs	Lexicon style Pharmacological	Malayalam
12	Sannipāta chikitsa		Treatment of sannipāta	
13	Aṣṭāṅgaśarīra	Vaidyaratnam P.S. Varier	Ayurvedic Anatomy	Sanskrit

14	Bṛhat Sarīra	,,	Anatomy	Sanskrit
15	Sodhanacikitsā	Manakkodam Ksavan Vaidyar	Pañcakarma	Manipravalam
16	Prayogasamuccaya	Kochunni thampuran	Toxicology	Manipravālam
17	Viṣavaidyajyotsnikā	Karattu Namboothori	Toxicology	Manipravālam
18	Ārogyacintāmaṇi	Vallathol Narayana Menon	Pediatrics	Malayalam
19	Sarvagarala pramocana	Kuttamath Cheriya Rama Kurup	Toxicology	Malayalam
20	Rasopaniṣat	Unknown	Rasaśāstra (medicinal application of metals and minerals)	Sanskrit
21	Arogyakalpadruma	Rama Varier Kaikkulangara	Pediatrics	Sanskrit

Lost textbooks (Luptatantras)

Although we have rich tradition of textbooks in Āyurveda available now, that much of the textbooks are believed to have been lost in different turns of history due to various reasons. Some of them were lost completely; some, partially. Many masters who were contemporary to the authors of greater triad wrote their own textbooks. Textbooks like *Agniveśasaṃhitā* (the original version of *Carakasaṃhitā*), *Vṛddhasauśruta* (original version of *Suśrutasaṃhitā*), etc. were lost after their redaction as *Carakasaṃhitā* and *Suśrutasaṃhitā* respectively. There is a reference in *Suśrutasaṃhitā*[7] about Brahmasaṇhitā, the first textbook of Āyurveda, consisting of thousand chapters and one lakh ślokas; but, the book was never referred to by any master in a later period.

Commentators like Cakrapāṅidatta, Vijayarakṣita, Śrīkanṭha, Indu, etc. quoted richly from textbooks which were lost afterwards (see table-8). Many of the lost textbooks have the above references as the sole evidence for their existence. The missing of such texts might have been happened due to many reasons like lack of preservation, lack of popularity, their similarity with famous textbooks etc.

Table–8: Lost textbooks (luptatantras)

Sl	Name of text	Author	Quoted by	Content	Relation with No.
book				other texts	
1	Agnivesāsaṃhitā	Agniveśa	Cakrapāṇi, Vijayarakṣita	General medicine Carakasaṃhitā	Original text of
2	Añjananidāna	Agniveśa	—	Pathology	—
3	Jatūkarṇasaṃhita	Jatūkarna	Cakrapāṇi, Vijayarakṣita	General medicine	Similarity with Agniveśasaṃhitā
4	Parāśarasaṃhitā	Parāśara	Cakrapāṇi, Vijayarakṣita	General medicine	Similarity with Agniveśasaṃhitā
5	Kshārapānisaṃhitā	Kṣārapāṇi	Cakrapāṇi, Vijayarakṣita	General medicine	Similarity with Agniveśasaṃhitā
6	Kharanādasaṃhitā	Kharanāda	Hemādri, Vijayarakshita	—	—
7	Viśvāmitrasaṃhitā	Viśvāmitra	Cakrapāṇi, Sivadasasen	—	—
8	Agastyasaṃhitā	Agastya	—	Paediatrics	Similar to Kāśyapasaṃhitā
9	Aupadhenavatantra	Aupadhenava	Dalhana	Surgery Suśrutasaṃhitā	Similar to
10	Aurabhratantra	Aurabhra	Dalhana	Surgery Suśrutasaṃhitā	Similar to
11	Vṛddhasuśrutatantra	Vṛddhasuśruta	Vijayarakṣita, Srīkanṭha	Different from	original Suśrutasaṃhitā
12	Pauṣkalāvatatantra	Pauṣkalāvata	Cakrapāṇi	Surgery	Similar to Suśruta
13	Vaitaranatantra	Vaitarana	Dalhana	Surgery	Similar to Suśruta
14	Bhojatantra	Bhoja			
15	Bhālukītantra	Bhalukī			
16	Videhatantra	Videha	Dalhana	Ophthalmology	
17	Nimitantra	Nimi	Dalhana	Ophthalmology	
18	Karālatantra	Karāla	Dalhana	Ophthalmology	
19	Pārvatakatantra	Parvataka	Dalhana	Paediatrics	Similar to Kāśyapasaṃhitā
20	Kāśyapasaṃhitā	Kaśayapa	Dalhana, Cakrapāṇi	Toxicology	
21	Ālambāyanasaṃhitā	ālambāyana	Dalhana, Cakrapāṇi	Toxicology	
22	Uśanasaṃhitā	Uśana	Dalhana, Cakrapāṇi	Toxicology	
23	Lātyāyanasaṃhitā	Lātyāyana	Dalhana, Cakrapāṇi	Toxicology	

TEXTBOOKS IN MODERN AGE

After the medieval period, set back of Āyurveda happened due to the arrival of modern medicine. The trends of Āyurveda in this period can be represented as follows:

- Set back to Āyurveda by the invasion of Allopathic system and British rule
- Textbooks tried to incorporate modern knowledge prevalent then
- In the education there was a great transition from 'Gurukula' system to Institution system which made ample development in many ways. This change was associated with a paradigm shift from textbook study to syllabus oriented study
- After independence, ample efforts were not made to renovate Āyurveda in its natural form.
- All the above changes reflected in the nature and content of textbooks

Textbooks/Publications

The main textbooks published in this period showed a transition from pure Āyurveda by nominally incorporating modern principles. Among these texts, *Bhaiṣajyaratnāvalī* (written by Govindadas) and *Yogaratnākara* (author unknown) stood outstanding by way of presenting themselves in the form of classical texts in content and structure. They elaborated almost all the branches of Āyurveda including later developments like Rasaśāstra. The drug formulations explained in these texts became very popular in practice and manufacturing thereafter. Textbooks like *Siddhāntanidāna* and *Pratyakṣaśārīra* (both written by Gananāth Sen) made attempts to incorporate modern knowledge with Ayurvedic description in pathology and anatomy respectively. Vaidyaratnam P.S. Varier wrote *Bṛhacchārīra* and *Aṣṭāṅgaśārīra* in a view to make a compact textbook for learning Anatomy incorporating relevant portions from Āyurveda and modern anatomy, purely in Sanskrit. Commentaries for classic texts written in Hindi and other regional languages by various masters made learning of Āyurveda easy. Textbooks on Rasaśāstra like *Rasajalanidhi* (by Bhudev Mukherjee) tried to update the knowledge in the field.

Another major turn in this period was the renovation and publication of the manuscript of the *Kāṣyapasaṃhitā*, which was thought to be lost, by the Rajaguru of Nepal, Pt. Hemarājaśarmā in 1890's. He wrote an elaborate introduction (*upodghāta*) to this text which is now considered as an authentic document of the history of Āyurveda.

Other advancements in the modern age in the sector of publication can be abridged as follows:

- Publication of Journals
- Subject specific publications by various Institutions
- Research Publications
- Pharmacopoea
- Syllabus oriented text books
- Textbooks for public education

Conclusion

While examining the Textbook tradition of Āyurveda, it is obvious that the wealth of literature in Āyurveda is contributed by many masters at various levels of its development. Unlike other forms of creative literature, scientific literature needs updating and editing to a greater extent. In Āyurveda, there was a rich tradition in the above regards, but, essentially there were ups and downs in the whole scenario. From all above, we can readily reach in a conclusion that a scientific textbook is not a product, but, a process which is still on its track.

References

1. *Suśrutasaṃhitā,* Sūtrasthāna 1.6; Carakasaṃhitā Sutrasthāna, 30.20.
2. Commentary on *Carakasaṃhitā,* Sūtrasthāna 1.2, by Cakrapāṇidatta
3. *Vistārayati leśoktam*
   sankṣipatyativistaram
   saṃskarāta kurute tantram
   purānam ca punarnavam
4. *Carakasaṃhitā,* Sūtrasthāna, 30. .31
5. *Carakasaṃhitā,* Vimānasthāna, 8.3.
6. Commentary on *Aṣṭāṅgahṛdaya,* Uttarasthāna, 40.80, by Arunadatta.
7. *Suśrutasaṃhitā,* Sūtrasthāna, 1.6.

Bibliography

1. *Āyurvedacaritram* (Malayalam), Dr. N.V. Krishnankutty Varier, Kottakkal Āyurveda Series:24, Publication Division, Aryavaidyasala, Kottakkal, 3rd revised ed., 2002.
2. Vāgbhaṭa, *Aṣṭāṅgahṛdayu,* With Commentaries of Arunadatta and Hemādri, Jaikrishnadas Āyurveda Series (no.52), Chaukhabha Orientalia, Varanasi, Ninth Edition 2005.
3. Caraka *Carakasaṃhitā,* Krishnadas Āyurveda Series 66, with commentary by Chakrapānidatta, Krishnadas Academy Varanasi, 2000.
4. Suśruta *Śuśrutasaṃhitā,* Jaikrishnadas Āyurveda Series, 34, with commentary by Dalhaṇa, Varanasi, Chaukhambha Orientalia, Varanasi, 8th ed., 2005.
5. Nīlamegha *Tantrayuktivicāra,* edited by Prof. N. Muthuswāmy, Publication Division, Govt. Āyurveda College, Thiruvananthapuram, 1976

15

Toxicology in Āyurveda

N. Sam

Toxicology is an important branch of Āyurveda. The ancient traditional Āyurveda practioners recorded their knowledge, case diaries and practical experiences in palmleaf manuscripts. The Oriental Research Institute and Manuscripts Library in its collection 162 manuscripts related to Toxicology. Multiple copies are available for certain works like *Jyotsnikā, Dūtalakṣaṇa, Lakṣaṇāmṛta, Viṣacikitsā, Viṣacandrikā, Viṣanārayaṇīya, Viśamocana, Viṣahara mantras* and medicines, etc. The content of these works are the origin of *nagās* (snakes), different kinds of snakes and its physiological features, special features and mannerisms of the messenger like their words, position and action, features related to time. i,e,, the day, week, lunar eclipse, etc., *tridoṣa* characteristics (three humours—*vāta, pitta, kapha*), peculiarities of the wound, spreading of the poison in *saptadhatus* (seven elements—skin, blood, flesh, fat, bone, bone marrow and semen), first aid for snake poison, symptoms and treatments for the poison of Cobra, Viper, Karivizhala, Venthiran and Water snakes, life saving medicines and other medicines for eradicating snake poison, etc. In addition to snake poison descriptions are there for the treatment of rat poison, spider poison, biting of mad dogs, cat, scorpion, monkey, wolf, horse, man, frog, fish, etc.

The works start with the description of the origin of serpants. In the beginning there were eight serpants (Aṣṭanāgas) namly, Ananta, Vaśuki, Takṣaka, Karkkoḍaka, Padma, Mahārāja, Saṅkhapāla and Gulika. They were the sons of Agni, Indra, Vāyu and Varuṇa. Śeṣa (Ananta) and Gulika were the sons of Agni and they belonged to the Brāhmaṇa jāti with Agni varṇa. Vāsuki and Saṅkhapāla were the sons of Indra with yellow colour and they are considered as royal serpents (Kṣatriya vaṃśa). Takṣaka and Mahāpadma were the sons of Vāyu; they belonged to Vaiśyājāti and are black in colour. Padma and Karkkoḍaka belonged to Śūdrajāti and were the sons of Varuṇa. They are white in colour. Ananta Serpent have 1000 heads, Vāsuki and Saṅkhapala have 800 heads each, Takṣaka and Mahāpadma have 500 heads each and Padman and Karkkodaka have 300 heads each. The other serpants are considered to be the descendents of these Aśṭānāgas. Cobra, Viper, Rajila are the common varieties and Venthiran is a cross bread or mixed variety. There are twenty-six varities of Cobra, sixteen varieties of Viper, thirteen varities of Rajilam and twenty-one varieties of Viyanthiran.

Cobra poison will create pain and it is of *Vāta prakṛti*. Viper poison will creat burning sensation and it is of *pitta prakṛti*. Rajila poison will create bulging in the wound and it is of *kapha prakṛti*. Venthiran is of mixed nature.

Spreading of Poison

The diagnosis of different types of poisons are made by observing the symptoms of the wounds and also of the patient. When a person is affected with snake poison, at the first stage it exists only in the skin for 100 *mātrās*. When the poison exists in the skin the hair of the patient will stand on end. When it passes on to the blood the patient will sweat. Then it enter into the flesh and the patient will feel hot. As the poison enters into the fat (medas) the patient will vomit and shiver. Then it passes on to the bone. At this stage the patient could not see anything and the neck will get choked. When the poison enters into bone-marrow hiccup will occur and the patient will take deep-breath. At last the poison will enter into the semen, then the patient gets faint and will die. At each stage there are different kinds of medicines to treat the patient. By observing the symptoms the physician could diagnose the positions of the poison and could prescribe the medicine accordingly.

Aśvagandhā (Amukkuram) is very effective for eradicating cobra poison. Sandal (Candana) for Viper, Ginger for Karivizhala are also very effective for eradication. As Viyanthiran (venthiran) is a cross variety, the above said medicines are mixed up together and given to the patient for its eradication. For rat poison, Muthanga, Madhujīrakam and Velladampu are very effective. These medicines are crushed with milk and can be pasted all over the body, then given for drinking. Water should be poured over head (dhārā) without any break. This will eradicate almost all kinds of snake poisons. *Nasya, pāna, lepa,* and *dhārā* with certain medicines are the processes for the eradication of toxicity. First aid for snake poison and specific medicines are also prescribed for each symptom.

16

Uses of Herbal Medicine

P. PREMA

Today in this modern world competing with the advancement of Science, diseases are increasing day by day in lightning speed and the disappointed people are also going behind fancy advertisements for cure of their ailments. Even for a slight headache people are in a fix to take a handful of tablets. The food habits, poluted atmosphere, nature of the work they do and the life style of the people has very much created a threat to the people about their health fearing what will happen tomorrow. But the palmleaf manuscripts in fact can give answer for many of the ailments, the society face today.

Palmleaf manuscripts are the heritage of our ancient culture. The manuscripts provide valuable treasures about Indian traditional system of Medicine. They provide informations about various diseases, their symptoms and the medicines for the treatment. Herbs are the basic ingredients used in the Indian traditional system of medicine. As we all know herbs played a vital role as medicine in olden days. But gradually the usage of herbals are diminished in the society because the Vaidyas who practised this system could not earn money even for their living. And the interest of learning this system also is diminished even by their children or by their disciples.

Presently when we go through the medical manuscripts we can clearly find that the herbals which we consider to be the weeds, play a very important role curing various ailments of the people. The pity is that people are not aware of the usage of the herbals and unknowingly they are destroying them thinking that they are weeds. They were unable to identify the useful herbs around them. The herbal medicines are harmless and are without any side effects. According to the body condition there may be some unpleasant effects which can be treated very easily by another herb or combination of herbs.

Herbs can be used both internally and externally. They can be used singly or in combination with other herbs. A single drug obtained from the herbals can be utilized for various ailments when they are given with different *Anupānas,* i.e., mixing medium depending upon the *vāta, pitta* and *kapha* body conditions. A single herb also can be utilized for different ailments depending upon their usage.

In the Siddha system of medicine which is coming under the Indian traditional system of medicine there are thirty-two varieties of internal medicine and thirty-two of external medicine. Identification of particular herb is a very important aspect here. The unnoticed herbs which we consider to be the waste plants are the important ingredients which can cure our primitive as well as serious ailments. So it is our prime duty to refresh the society to gain at least a preliminary knowledge about these herbs and their usages. Even the herbal products in our kitchen are very simple remedies, which can prevent serious ailments.

In this article we will discuss about a few herbs which can be used by any one as simple remedies.

For migrane, headache: *Leucas aspera,* Family, *Labiatae.*

Five to ten drops of fresh juice of it with equal quantity of saline water used as nasal drops will relieve the pain in short duration.

For fever: *Andrographis paniculata.* Family—*Acanthaceae.*

Sixty grams of the fresh plant made into a decoction for three doses a day will relieve us from fever.

For Scorpion bite: *Solanum melongena,* Family—*Solanaceae.*

Cut a brinjal into two pieces. Tie one piece to the stinged place so that the cut end touches the body. After some time remove the piece and tie the other piece in the same way.

For eye (especially for contageous viral eye disease): *Cleome viscosa.* Family—*Capparidaceae.*

Crush the plant and put it inside a tumbler and keep the eyes facing that so that the volatile oil will act upon the eyes.

For removing dust from the eye: *Borreria hispida,* Family—*Rubiaceae.*

Take fresh root of this plant and chew it for 5 to 10 minutes.

For skin irritations or allergies by some other herbs or insects *Ocimum sanctum.* Family—*Labiatae.*

Take fresh juice and smear it on the body surface.

For cough with suffocation:

1. *Solanum trilobatum.* Family—*Solanaceae.*

Three to four fresh leaves eaten with an interval of 3 to 4 hours.

2. *Ocimum sanctum.* Family—*Labiatae.*

Coleus aromaticus. Family—*Lamiaceae.*

Take five to seven ocimum fresh leaves and then a single Coleus leaf.

For repeated vomiting: *Murraya koenigii,* Family—*Rutaceae.*

Roast fresh leaves (handful) then little salt and add one cup of water to it and make it a decoction as half cup and take internally.

For over bleeding: *Alysicarpus monilifer,* Family—*Leguminosae.*
Crush the plant and Keep it on the centre of the head.

For Rheumatic pain: *Tamarindus indicus,* Family—*Leguminosae.*
Fresh leaves along with little salt boiled with more water and do sponging.

For worms: *Aloe vera,* Family—*Liliaceae*
Take fresh fleshy leaf and eat the inner succulent portion in empty stomach for three days.

For fresh bruises: *Tridax procumbens,* Family—*Asteraceae*
Clean the surface and apply fresh juice of the leaves. Do not wet until the wound is healed.

For swellings because of trauma: *Azadirachta indica,* Family—*Meliaceae.*
Grind tender leaves into fine paste and apply it to the swellings.

For common cold: *Santalum album,* Family—*Santalaceae.*
Little powder rolled in a cotton cloth, burn and inhale the smoke.

For anaemia:
Murraya koenigii, Family—*Rutaceae.*
Moringa oleifera, Family—*Moringaceae.*
Allium cepa, Family—*Liliaceae.*
Thirty grams of the above three with five grams of *Cuminum cyminum,* Family—*Umbelliferae.*
Make a decoctions for fifteen days. Twice daily.

Hybanthus enneaspermus. Family—*violaceae.*

1. Fresh plant made into a paste applied to pimple will give quick remedy.
2. Fresh plant made into paste and applied to nerve dislocations created because of dislocation of bone joints.
3. Fresh juice two to three drops applied to the eye can cure many eye diseases.
4. Fresh plant (five gram) eaten daily for forty-one days increase the potency of men.
5. Fresh plant made into paste mixed with water applied to the head reduces dandruff.

Uncontrolled Urination due to geriatrics: *Tinospora cordifolia,* Family—*Menispermaceae*

Take three to four pieces of mature stem of one inch length, peel it and take internally to for one week strengthen the bladder.

Thus herbal medicines when rightly used can cure manyt ailments even today.

17

Varma as Therapy

T. MOHANA RAJ

Varma is a special branch of subject coming under the Siddha syste of medicine, which is called as the Tamil Traditional Medicine formed by the ancient Siddhars. In olden days *Varma* was mainly used in martial arts. It was also used as a therapy by a group of people, i.e., the palmirah climbers. As per Varma therapy there are 108 main *Varma* points in our body. The word Varma is also known as *Kāla, Vasi, Yoga, Uyir, Jīvan, Prāṇa,* etc. The word *Prāṇa* and *Jīvana* referes to cosmic energy into the vital air—the essential life force. We can feel the Varma points through the sense of touch but they are invisible to the naked eye. Varma therapy cures nervous disorders and resultant symptoms due to trauma by stimulating some other therapeutic points known as *Adankals*.

The Varmas are inconspicuous and hence they are kept secret. Varmas are points where we feel the presence of the *prāṇa*; (life), hence they are fatal points. According to the Siddhars in human body are there 72,000, blood vessels and the *prāṇa* is circulating along with the blood through them. When a trauma occurs to this circulating vessel in particular points with a specific force, paralysis, formation of some diseases, unconsciousness, or death may occur. Therapeutically the *Adankals* are used to treat the impact of Varma. If the effect of trauma is not reversed within a stipulated time, it may become fatal also.

When a person learns about the Varma points he is forced to learn about the *Adankals* because the impact of Varma can be reversed or treated only by stimulating the *Adankals* if not one has to face unpleasant situations.

The science of Varma is developed in school of martial arts known as Silambam, Kalari, Adimurai, etc. During fight between two or more persons by striking a particular Varma with force, the enemy can be paralyzed or made unconscious for the time being. Even today the study of Varma is important in schools of martial arts for Kalari/Adimurai for self defense

"Ullapadi Nootiyettu thala chavahum
Unarvahi aththalangal uyirumahum
Kallamutta aththalangal piniyumahum
Kalangamattal aththalangal sugame kanum
Ullunarvāi aththalangal vasiyetta
Uttathinal aththalangal uruthi serum
Pulladi pol aththalangal kandavargal
Pugalargal elloru puviyulloke"

According to the Siddhars there are 108 Varma points in our human body. These 108 points are capable of killing a person, make him diseased, or healthy or they can make him to continue his life span.

Origin of Varma

The first Siddhar Lord Śiva taught Varma to his son Lord Muruga and Lord Muruga, taught this to his disciple Agastya and Agastya in turn taught this to his disciples and so on. Agastya is considered to be an important Siddhar by all. He was also called as 'Kumbamuni'. He along with his disciples 'Theriar' composed Varma books. Agastya staying in the 'Pothigai' mountain region developed Tamil Siddha Medicine and also Varma medicine.

Bohar is also a Siddhar who is a disciple of Kālangi; they together composed Varma books. There is a belief among the people, that Bohar made a statue for 'Palni Murugan' which is made with an alloy of nine minerals (*Nava pashana—Kattu*). So it is understood that Bohar also is a Siddhar who had reverence to the ancestoral Siddhar Lord Muruga. So Lord Śiva, Lord Muruga. Agastya, Kālangi, Bohar, Pulipani are few persons who are given importance while we talk about Varma.

Growth of Varma in Kanyakumari District

The Copper plate document obtained from Parthipasekarapura (Parthipapuram) which is nearer to Munchirai of Kanyakumai district in Tamil Nadu State, says that in the ninth Century AD. (857-85) there reigned a Shepherd race king Koharunanthadakkan who built a city Parthipapura and constructed a temple and a University. In that University the Varma and other martial arts were taught.

Some reasons for the downfall of Varma medicine

Varma, a special branch of science which is flourished in the Kanyakumari District is not popular in other places. In this District, still this branch is learnt in 'Guru-Śiṣya' tradition or in traditional discipleship. But the downfall of the Varma practice creates some different reactions.

The people who know these techniques were not ready to give the knowledge to the public. Because the Gurus teach the disciples that they will be cursed and punished if they give this to an improper person. Because this art can kill a person with a finger or two without anyone's knowledge. So if it reaches to an improper person he will misuse this knowledge which is irreparable. And for the fear of being cursed the diciples concealed this knowledge. Now-a-days there are not sufficient number of disciples to follow the Varma therapy.

Qualities of a Varma desciple

A disciple who wants to learn Varma must have a control over sexual feelings and anger. He must be pious and respect his teacher, he should control himself, must have good concentration, should not have a wavering mind.

> *"Muduhuvathu sandala kobathale*
> *Munparan pinparan muraigal paran*
> *Kaduhuvathu āngara mathil kondu*
> *Katta vithaiathai mathil enni*
> *Naduhuvathu naloor perioor thamai*
> *Nanilathil elaikalai nadunga seithu*
> *Kodugava eedu seithu kolvanappa*
> *Kodumpava avanai vanthu kurugu thane".*

The above poetry says that only this knowledge can be given to God-fearing people and if it is given to others the donor will be sent to hell.

How Varma is Occuring

Hit by a stout stick or some pointed objects, by hands, by a fall from a height, breakages etc. the created trauma causes Varma injury when it affects the Varma points.

Varma–108

Totally 108 Varma points were identified by the Siddhars in our body. They are Classified as "PaduVarma 12" and "ThodVarma 96". They are further classified as, in head 25, neck to the umbilicus–45, umbilicus to the anus 9, in hand–14, in leg 15.

'PaduVarma' means that if the trauma occurs in the correct 'mātrā'; (force) there is more chance of death to the injured.

'ThoduVarma' is not so dangerous like PaduVarma but it may be fatal. Usually it will paralyse or will create some disorders.

Varma points in the head

(1). Kondaikolli Varma; (2) Seerumkolli Varma; (3) Pidari Varma; (4) Suruthi Varma; (5) Porchai Varma; (6) Kutti Varma; (7) Sevikutti Varma; (8). Poigai Varma; (9) Natchathira Varma; (10) Kampoori Varma; (11) Mūrthi Varma; (12) Annan Varma; (13) Thilartha Varma; (14) Minvetti Varma; (15). Manthira Varma; (16) Nema Varma; (17) Patchi Varma; (18) Kannadi Varma; (19) Pala Varma; (20) Kona Varma; (21) Uthira Varma; (22) Ottu Varma; (23) Urakka Varma; (24) Sanguthiri Varma; (25) Sumai Varma.

Varma points between neck and umbilicus

(1) Kakattai Varma; (2) Kathir Varma; (3) Kama Varma; (4) Puthi Varma; (5) Sakthi Varma; (6) Thivalai Varma; (7) Eanthi Varma; (8) Piratharai Varma; (9) Kuthu Varma; (10) Ulputta Varma; (11) Mari Varma; (12) Amathu Varma; (13) Munkamunthan Varma; (14) Kanthari Varma; (15) Athi kanthari Varma; (16) Thūsiga Varma; (17) Asta Varma; (18) Koombu Varma; (19) Ner Varma (20) Urumi Varma; (21) Adappa Varma; (22) Mundellu Varma; (23) Periya Athisurukki Varma; (24) Siriya Ahisurikki Varma; (25) Mun surithi Varma; (26) Pin surithi Varma; (27) Pallai Varma; (28) Udal surukki Varma 29) Kareeral Varma; (30) Veleeral Varma; (31) Thumpi Varma; (32) Kaiketti Varma; (33) Sadapira Varma; (34) Kilipira Varma; (35) Kilimega Varma; (36) Puya Varma; (37) Vilangu Varma; (38) Suliyadi Varma; (39) Sulikki Varma; (40) Poonool Varma; (41) Natellu Varma; (42) Katchai Varma; (43) Kaikottu Varma; (44) Vaiyu Varma; (45) Anna Varma.

Varma points between umbilicus and anus

(1) Mūthira Varma; (2) Kalladai Varmam: (3) Valampuri Varma; (4) Edampuri Varma; (5) Vellurumi Varma; (6) Vallurumi Varma; (7) Narankutti Varma; (8) Ani Varmam: (9) Ānthai Varmam.

Varma points in the hand

(1) Mozhi Varma; (2) Thetchanai Varma; (3) Soondothari Varma; (4) Chundothari Varma; (5) Vellai Varma; (6) Kavali Varma; (7) Manipantha Varma; (8) Ānthai Varma; (9) Visamanipantha Varma; (10) Mudakku Varma; (11) Muttu Varma; (12) Mundakathu Varma; (13) Kaisulukku Varma; (14) Asaivu Varma.

Varma points in the leg

(1) Kalvellai Varma; (2) Uppukutti Varma; (3) Kuttikai Varma; (4) Viruthi Varma; (5) Soondathati Varma; (6) Pada Varma; (7) Kannupugai Varma; (8) Kuthikal Varma; (9) Viguthi Varma; (10) Kuthiraimuga Varma; (11) Komberi Varma; (12) Konasanni Varma; (13) Kalmuttu Varma; (14) Kāri Varma; (15) Urumi Varma.

Injury to Varmas are immediately treated by stimulating certain other related *Adankal.* i.e., after a forced trauma or Varma, to safeguard the life of the injured, some immediate massage techniques are adopted. Some special massage techniques are applied to certain related Varmas along with pressure, striking, tapping, rubbing, shaking, fondling and squeezing with the palm and fingers which is known as *'Adankal'*. Ilakkumurai and Adankal (corrective treatment) is a technique used by manipulation and stimulation of some other Varmas by the above said special massage techniques. After regaining consciousness, the person should undergo special massage. There is internal medicine for trauma to each Varma and also as per the symptoms of the injured. The massage is done by specially trained persons by expertly moving the palms over the body after applying oil with varying degree of force. Different methods of massage are being done for curing different Varma injuries.

This valuable art must be popularized among the medical experts thereby preventing unnecessary death and paralysis of organs.

18

Vikṛti Vijñjāna-Samkṣepa: Impish Knowledge-Concise

SARAMMA VARGHESE

Various traditional branches of medical science existed since much before the onset and development of modern branches of medical science. Āyurveda system of medical science, which developed much later, has received seminal contributions from these traditional branches of medical sciences. Detecting the disease merely by reading the symptoms, diagnosing the disease by assessing the pulse rate, *sveda, virecana, vamana, uzhichil,* etc. are some of the methods of these traditional methods of treatment.

Āyurveda has divided all the elements of the human body into three categories namely *doṣas* (bad things), *dhātus* (minerals) and *malangal* (excreta). The knowledge ('vijñānam') of mischief making (*vikṛti*) of these three elements in an Ayurvedic pattern is known as Impish Knowledge (*vikṛti vijñāna*). Since the intention of both the *vaidya* (Āyurveda doctor) and the *rogī* (patient) is to cure the *vikṛti* (trouble) caused to the body and restore its normalcy, the awareness of *vikṛti vijñāna* (impish knowledge) is equally vital for both the doctor and the patient.

We can understand *vikṛti vijñāna* (impish knowledge) only by relating it to health and in a relative fashion. So before considering the painful troubles caused, we need to have an understanding of the precise symptoms of health. Ācārya Suśruta has exquisitely pointed out the following symptoms of health: the balance or state of equlibrium in the actions of the bodily elements *doṣa, dhātu, mala, agni* (Fire) and the consciousness of well-being , i.e. the happy state of soul, mind and the senses. It is worthy to note here the fact that no other branch of medical science defines health in such a balanced or holistic fashion (the word used in Sanskrit is *samyak* which cannot be translated into English—the dimensions of the word go beyond the dimensions of translation).

The *Vikṛti-vijñāna-samkṣepa* (impish knowledge-concise) deals with the prediction of the days remaining for a person's demise, chiefly by reading the symptoms of the disease. The paper has been prepared on the basis of the manuscripts Thaliyolas preserved and kept tagged with the register numbers 10985-E, 10955-C, and 5791-B in the Manuscripts Library of the University of Kerala.

Constitution of the Grantha (Book)

The work starts with a benediction to God as seen in most other *Granthas* of this kind. The symptoms arising out of the changes occurring in shape, colour, sound, action and the five senses proclaim the day of death. Key facts like the name of the author (Sri Ramadasan) and that the manuscripts are multilingual are evidently inscribed in *Grantha* 10985-E.

Contents

The work starts by showing the changes occurring in the five senses:

> *Eyes*: If the eyes move fast and stops, bulges, then draws inward, narrows, then expands and if they are red like those of a dove, or like those of a fire-brand, with eyebrows bent and bow-shaped, and to looking a dazed manner as if nothing can be seen, and moreover if there is a dripping

or tears oozing out, then death is sure to happen.

Nose: The nostrils expanding, pimples surfacing out of small swellings, bursting and getting worn out on the nose and weakening it are collectively an indicator of death. *Tongue*: The left-prone twisting of the tongue, perhaps growing and parching and then not knowing the tastes, feeling a numbness, feeling the prick of a thorn, darkening and increasing in size, feeling the uneasiness of something pasted to it, speaks largely of an impending death that is certain.

Ears: Death is sure if clouds, conches, musical instruments, like *vīṇā*, kuzhal(flute) etc. are heard when they are not producing sounds, and not heard when they are really producing sounds. When one closes ears with hands because of jarring sound from inside and along with it when the tongue looses its discretion for tastes, and then the nose losing the capability to sense the stench of wick burning without any oil are sure signs of death.

Skin: Death is sure to take place in six days' span when the body after a dip, like the leaf of a lotus plant, feels zero wetness or touch of water. If the vein on the body turns turmeric yellow, gleaming dust accumulates on the eyebrow and smoke-like thin air rises from atop the head the healthy will be dead in six days and the unhealthy in three days, time.

Lips: If the lowerlip curves downwards and the upperlip curves upwards, and both the lips acquire a vivid dark reddish purple colour of a Njara fruit death is sure to occur.

Teeth: If the teeth is covered with decay-moss, turns black and dark, as if mud-smeared, and if one by one teeth ejects out without any reason, death is sure to occur.

Veins: If the veins become clearly visible on the forehead and the rest of the body unlike they were in yesteryears death is sure in six months.

Body Parts: Numbness of real physical pain, shape-alteration and the body acquiring a brownish hue, feeling of coldness just after sweating, feeling of vigour just after depression, sneezing and coughing with a strange change of sound are all signs of death.

Breath: If one struggles to breathe, and if the breath smells, and if the taste of such breath draws in flies and ants death is sure to occur.

Body: Unprecedented ups and downs in body temperature, sweating even after cooling the body, feeling cold in the bosom while feeling a rise in temperature in the stomach, feeling thirsty after emptying the bowels, and if all the excreta ejects out together death is sure.

Sight: Seeing sky as earth and earth as sky, brightness as darkness and darkness as brightness, wind as fire, varied colours having the blackness of discontent, seeing several moons, and without any black spots on it augurs death.

Sound: If the sound lowers, and one speaks the never intended, body losing vitality, sound reflecting the depression of the mind, always complaining, death is sure to occur next morning itself.

Death is sure to occur if the legs get bowed because of falling down, body losing energy even after consuming food, occurrence of dysentery even after mild intake of food etc. Death will occur easily for the diseased and it will occur in a delayed fashion to the healthy if the aforementioned symptoms are sighted.

The diseases that commonly occur in the ancient times

are mentioned: *jvara* (fever), *raktapita* (tuberculosis), piles, dysentery, pressure, swellings, stomach ailments, *pāṇḍu roga,* respiratory ailments, etc. Their symptoms, seen from the changing features of the body are detailed. Diseases are of two kinds: one that leads to death and the other that will be cured if treated in the right manner. The *Vikṛti-vijnāna-śamkṣepa* reveals precise ideas about those diseases which lead to death (determined through the various signs of illness suffered by the patient); it also details the patient's longevity. The changes in shape, body, colour, sound, actions, five senses etc. are closely observed and the time of death is determined with the aid of the ideas inferred from an assessment of these changes.

All the medical sciences existing in various forms in various parts of the world deal with the nature and symptoms of *vikṛti* (ailment) and *svāsthya* (health) according to the kind of logic described in each of them and hence each one is unique. The ultimate aim of all medical sciences is health preservation but the way of treatment devised for it is different in each case.

Vikṛti(ailment) manifests itself generally through strange signs and symptoms. During the time of diagnosis based on the conditions and features specified the causes of an ailment have to be found out. A skilful Vaidya doctor should have an indepth and precise knowledge of '*vikṛti vijñāna*' which in the cases of specific diseases needs various experi-mentation and analyses to find out the signs symptomatic of each disease. Ācārya Suśruta has identified six stages for *Vikṛti*: *Cayam, Prakopa, Prasāra, Sthāna Samṣraya, Vyakti* and *Bheda.* According to Suśrutha, *Vikṛti* appears in its real form in the stage of *Sthāna Saṃśraya* and so it is the most important phase. Since it is easier and effective for modern medical science to diagnose and find curative methods of treatment through various experiments with diseases *Vikṛti Vijñāna-Saṃkṣepa* becomes inevitable for the study of medicine..

References

1. *Pracheena Kairaly*, vol. 26, ORI and MSS Library, University of Kerala, 1992.
2. Aṣṭāṅgahṛdaya

Contributors

1.	N.P.P. Namboothiri	:	Sreedhariyam Ayurvedic Eye Hospital and Research Centre, Koothattukulam.
2.	P.R. Jaya	:	Medical Officer, Govt. Ayurveda Dispensary, TVM.
3.	Rejani, R.S	:	Asst. Professor, ORIML, University of Kerala.
4.	R. Girija	:	Asso. Professor (Rtd), ORIML, University of Kerala.
5.	Lalu S Kurup	:	Senior Research Fellow, ORIML, University of Kerala.
6.	K. Muthulekshmi	:	Asst. Professor, Department of Vedanta, Sree Sankaracharya University of Sanskrit, TVM.
7.	P.L Shaji	:	Manuscript Conservator, ORIML, University of Kerala.
8.	K.G Sreelekha	:	Professor & Head, ORIML, University of Kerala.
9.	Radha	:	Research Scholar, ORIML, University of Kerala.
10.	Senthil, N.	:	Research Scholar, ORIML, University of Kerala.

11.	P. Vasumathy Devi	: Asso. Professor (Rtd), Department of History, University of Kerala.
12.	S.A.S. Sarma	: EFEO, 19, Dumas Street, Pondicherry.
13.	O. Padmakumari	: Asst. Professor, ORIML, University of Kerala.
14.	Vinod Kumar, M.V	: Asso. Professor, V.P.S.V Ayurveda College, Kottakkal.
15.	N. Sam	: Professor (Rtd), ORIML, University of Kerala.
16.	P. Prema	: Vice Principal/HOD, ATSVS Sidha Medical College & Hospital, Munchirai, K.K District.
17.	T. Mohana Raj	: Akhila Thiruvithamcode Sidha Vaidya Sangam, K.K District.
18.	Saramma Varghese	: Lecturer, Department of Malayalam, St. Thomas College, Kozhenchery.